Vinegar Prescription
by Emily Thacker

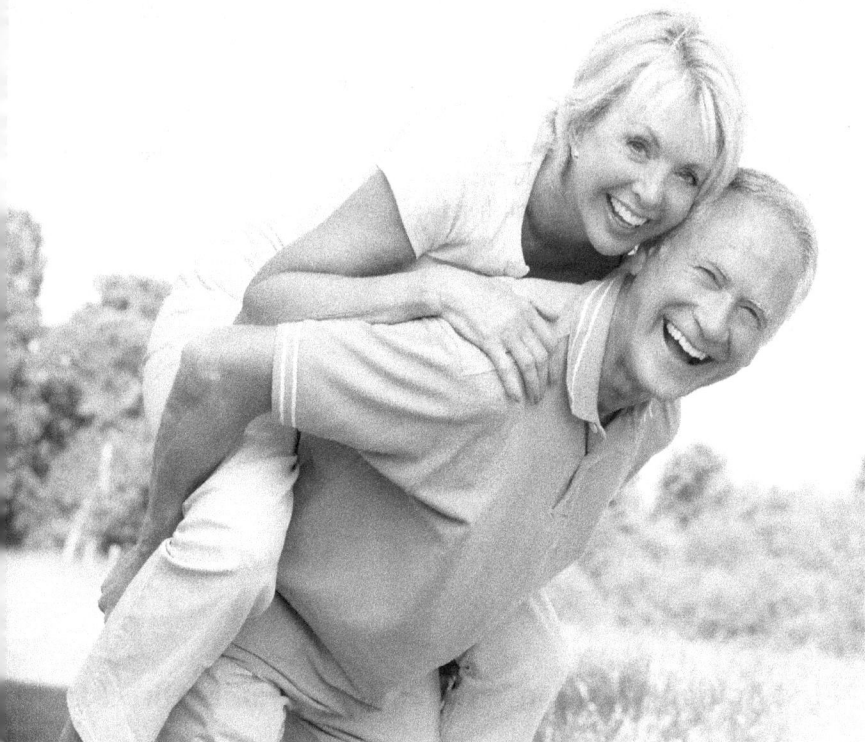

Published by:

James Direct Inc

500 S. Prospect Ave.

Hartville, Ohio 44632

U.S.A.

This book is intended as a record of folklore and historical solutions and is composed of tips, suggestions, and remembrances. It is sold with the understanding that the publisher is not engaged in rendering medical advice and does not intend this as a substitute for medical care by qualified professionals. No claims are intended as to the safety, or endorsing the effectiveness, of any of the remedies which have been included and the publisher cannot guarantee the accuracy or usefulness of individual remedies in this collection.

If you have a medical problem you should consult a physician.

Not For Resale

ISBN: 978-1-62397-079-6

Printing 12 11 10 9 8 7 6 5 4 3 2 1

First Edition   **Copyright 2018**   **James Direct Inc**

Table of Contents

Introduction
The Case for Vinegar

W hy a book about vinegar? The obesity rate in the United States stands at a staggering 35% - not including that percentage of the population considered merely "overweight." Diabetes is at an all-time high. Consumer costs for prescription medication is out of control, and the price of health insurance has skyrocketed. In short, healthcare in this country is at a tipping point.

The material presented in this book is meant to offer a better way, getting (returning) back to a simpler time when common (and not-so-common) health conditions were handled naturally. That is not to say this book is intended to negate everything modern medicine has to offer. Quite the contrary. Scientific research has led to some of the most remarkable medical discoveries ever imagined.

In the last 100 years alone, medical advances have paved the way to the discovery of insulin to help manage diabetes. We are no longer restricted to simple X-ray technology to "see" the un-seeable, but now regularly benefit from CT and MRI technology. Kidney dialysis and major organ replacement are no longer a fantastic idea, but a life-saving reality for millions. Fertility advances are commonplace, and infant mortality rates have plummeted. Surgical advances have led to shorter hospital stays. But perhaps the most innovative and pragmatic discovery has been the introduction of antibiotics which has revolutionized the way infections are treated.

And the newest of scientific breakthroughs are already on the horizon – everything from gene editing to cure disease to 3D prosthetic printing.

Advances Come With a Price

This book is not a repudiation of all things medical. Not at all. But it does some with the acknowledgment that along with these medical advances comes a sometimes-heavy price tag. For example, contemporary pharmaceutical medications, while more potent and widely prescribed than ever before come with risky potential side effects which must be considered when taking them. Just a few of these include:

- drug interactions
- addictions and dependency
- exorbitant costs
- overly taxing on liver and kidneys

Keep in mind neither prescribed or over the counter medications possess the ability to target only the afflicted area. Instead, the user is being subjected to these medications system-wide with oftentimes unintended consequences. In addition, long-term use can not only be taxing on the body itself, but also runs the risk of building up resistance to the drug, thus limiting future effectiveness.

Truth be told, many medications which are being currently prescribed have not been on the market long enough to adequately document the long-term effects on the body. Worse still, the majority of prescribed drugs merely mask the symptoms of an illness anyway, rather than treating its root cause.

It is past time we took seriously the effects these drugs have on our bodies. The ugly truth is that the majority of reasons doctors prescribe most medications could have been avoided by having made different lifestyle choices.

Because side effects associated with these medications can intensify over time and become riskier, one might do well to treat as many of these conditions naturally wherever possible, saving the more hardcore treatments for times they are most needed. You will find your body will become more healthy and resilient by improving its immune system, and, for those times when pharmaceutical drugs are the only path to wellness, your body will react better having not yet built up a tolerance or resistance to its use.

But this phenomenon is not limited to merely healthcare. The same applies to much of daily living, including a subject as seemingly benign as modern cleaning products.

At any given time, we can find literally hundreds of commercially-manufactured cleaning products on store shelves - with a "special" cleaning product available for every application imaginable. A cleaning solution formulated specifically for that porcelain toilet, but another for stainless steel faucets. Different products to choose from depending on the type of flooring: carpet, wood, tile, linoleum. Cleaning products for laundry, wood furniture, dishes, countertops (you wouldn't want to use that product made for solid surface on your granite countertops, would you?)

But what is the one trait they all share? Each is produced using chemicals you might not otherwise feel comfortable introducing into your home. Yet, we have come to rely on these chemicals every day – with each use having the potential of leaving behind sometimes toxic residue we continue to encounter long after. And, we have not begun to mention the production, application and disposal of these products which eventually find their way into streams and landfills.

It is now commonplace to find antibacterial additives in soaps and cleaning products. Research has shown these additions actually strengthen the resistance of antibiotic resistant bacteria, rending them more difficult to ultimately eliminate.

And that brings us to the purpose of this book – offering a realistic, natural alternative to sometimes unnecessary health solutions (when choosing the way we run our lives). Simply put, allowing you to become the driving force of your own health decisions.

The Vinegar Prescription lays out ways to introduce wholesome, all-natural vinegar into your lifestyle, offering a different perspective on better health. Why vinegar?

It might surprise you that vinegar contains much of the very same traits as so many of commercially manufactured entities we have discussed, but in a 100% natural form, and without any of the harmful side effects. These same illness-fighting characteristics sought in medications are found naturally and abundantly in everyday household vinegar:

- antibacterial
- antibiotic
- antiviral
- antifungal
- antimicrobial
- antiseptic
- antioxidant
- anti-inflammatory

Vinegar also boats a claim to fame that most drugs cannot. Scientific research studies have discovered that vinegar contains more than 90 different components or compounds with enormous health benefit to the human body. And, depending upon which type of vinegar is being used (apple cider versus white or distilled vinegar) an even more impressive list of essential vitamins, mineral and nutrients can be found:

- vitamin A and D
- vitamin B-6
- folate
- protein
- calcium
- iron
- fiber
- potassium
- carbohydrates
- folate
- ascorbic acid (vitamin C)
- thiamin (vitamin B-1)
- zinc
- riboflavin (vitamin B-2)
- niacin
- magnesium
- pantothenic acid

- copper
- phosphorus
- manganese
- tryptophan
- serine
- proline
- glycine
- glutamic acid
- aspartic acid
- alanine
- histidine
- phenylalanine
- arginine
- valine
- tyrosine
- cystine
- methionine
- lysine
- leucine
- threonine
- isoleucine

These crucial elements work in concert with the body's own immune system to not only fight disease and infection, but also build a healthier, stronger body – naturally.

All of these qualities add up to a dynamic substance, packed with elements the human body craves for proper function. Best of all, it is totally natural, with zero addictive qualities or unwanted side effects.

The Science Behind Vinegar

But this is really nothing new. Vinegar has been used for centuries to treat a variety of conditions, some through folklore and some handed down for generations with quite impressive results. And it seems science is now catching up to what some cultures have known for lifetimes, as healthcare institutions worldwide have worked vinegar into treatment protocol for a host of conditions.

Western Michigan University indicated vinegar can be used to increase the accuracy of conventional testing used to detect cervical cancer.

Ohio State University's hospital currently prescribes vinegar irrigation treatment for chronic inner ear infections, while the American Academy of Otolaryngology suggests a combination of vinegar and alcohol to care for swimmer's ear.

A research study conducted by the Journal of Diabetes Research shows vinegar can reduce hypoglycemia in patients suffering from type 2 diabetes.

The A.P. John Institute for Cancer Research has begun adding vinegar supplements to patient diets with the belief this treatment can help "shut off energy in cancer cells and cause them to die off."

Arizona State University details a research study in which participants took apple cider vinegar diluted in water with a saccharine additive and showed lower blood sugar levels following meals.

When post-surgery eye infections became problematic at Yale-New Haven Hospital, their Department of Bacteriology solved the issue by routinely cleaning scrub room sinks with a 1/2% solution of everyday household vinegar.

And these findings are not limited to the United States alone. Dr. Yoshio Takimo out of Japan's Shizuoka University determined vinegar helps maintain a healthy body and slows aging through the prevention of the formation of two fatty acids. This discovery deals with free radicals and cholesterol formations that can build up on the walls of blood vessels.

And this just begins to scratch the surface of vinegar's use in today's field of medicine. Amish households keep vinegar as a pantry staple for use in everything from cooking and home healing remedies to cleaning and gardening. Generations have used vinegar to treat sickness and promote better health.

The goal has remained the same as it has for centuries and in all walks of life: to live a happy, healthy life to its fullest. It is my true desire that the information in this book will help you achieve just that.

Happy Reading.

Chapter One
What is Vinegar?

Vinegar boasts a rich history as a medicinal cure, having been around nearly as long as civilization itself. Historical accounts detail a variety of vinegars found in ancient Rome prior to 1000 BC. It is repeatedly referred to in Biblical accounts, and archaeologists have identified vinegar residue in urn relics dating back to 3000 BC. Military armies throughout time, from the legendary armies of Rome to our own Civil War and World War 1 soldiers, used vinegar to strengthen the body and dress battlefield wounds.

Early physicians used vinegar and oils to immunize themselves from contracting the deadly black plague virus from their infected patients. One popular account being the legend of the four thieves who escaped the ravishes of the lethal disease by drinking garlic-infused vinegar – hence, today's Four Thieves Vinegar came to be known.

In what is possibly the most resounding endorsement for vinegar's healing capabilities comes from medicine's most esteemed alumni: Hippocrates himself, widely considered the father of modern medicine, regularly prescribed apple cider vinegar to treat a range of medical conditions in his own patients.

But what, exactly, is vinegar?

In a nutshell, vinegar is any alcoholic liquid that is allowed to ferment or sour. It is a solution comprised of water and acetic acid.

Vinegar is formed when a sugary liquid, like one made from pureed apples or even rice, is allowed to ferment into alcohol through a yeast reaction. Next, this newly formed alcoholic solution sours, and is changed yet again into an acetic acid solution.

Different types of vinegar

Vinegar is available in a variety of popular flavors, each with its own unique benefit. While the process of manufacturing vinegar remains basically the same for each, noticeable differences can be found in the end product. The manufacturing process of vinegar retains a good portion of the nutrients native to the original food from which it was made. This is particularly true of unpasteurized varieties. So it stands to reason the most important factor in determining which type of vinegar one uses lies in the original food used.

Let's take "simple" apple cider vinegar, for example. Apple cider vinegar is made from a variety of apples which are known to be high in healthful pectin, and contain more than 90 nutritional elements or compounds beneficial to the human body. So, when pureed apples are made into the final apple cider vinegar product, it retains the majority of these essential compounds, which translate into a highly useful and potent remedy for many health ailments. This transfer or continuation of nutrients accounts for the most obvious differences in the most popular types of vinegar.

Apple cider vinegar is one of the most popular vinegar varieties in the United States. It is made from different types of apples, and contains nutrients essential for good health, such as calcium, potassium, magnesium, copper, phosphorous and more. It also possesses enzymes as well as additional minerals and amino acids, making it an excellent choice for use in natural home health remedies.

White, or distilled, vinegar is manufactured through inexpensive product leftovers, such as corn. Due to its inexpensive cost, it is typically the preferred choice for cleaning, and is also the go-to vinegar for pickling and preserving the whiteness in light-colored foods, such as onions and cauliflower.

True **balsamic vinegar** is a rich, immensely-flavored vinegar hailing from the Modena region of Italy. It is a sweet wine vinegar, derived from the Trebbiano grape, aged in wooden storage barrels until it's vinegary tartness is overlaid with a sweet flavor. It tends to be an expensive choice, sometimes as costly as a good, aged wine, and is used in many culinary dishes worldwide.

Other vinegar varieties include wine, rice, champagne, malt, sherry and even vinegars infused with a near endless list of herbs.

Infused vinegars begin with its vinegar base and add various combinations of herbs and secondary foods, such as thyme, basil, tarragon, dill – basically any herb will work. Fruits can also be added, as well as the ever-popular garlic. Even edible flowers, like nasturtiums, can be found in infused vinegar. The rave of using an infused vinegar is found in the added health benefit that comes with whatever herb or food it has been infused with.

For example, garlic contains allicin, which is known to have potent medicinal benefits. It is also used to help lower blood pressure and reduce cholesterol levels. By infusion apple cider vinegar with garlic, one would receive the double health benefit of both foods in one combined solution. (Infused vinegars contain so much potentially beneficial attributes, we have dedicated an entire chapter to its use.)

Another overlooked aspect of vinegar is in the highly beneficial, yet unrefined, substance called "mother."

What is Mother of Vinegar?

Technically speaking, mother of vinegar is a substance formed during the fermentation process of liquid alcohol, and is made up of acetic acid bacteria and cellulose. In more practical terms, mother is the thick film or goop that can be found in unfiltered vinegar, usually the apple cider vinegar type, and can make vinegar appear cloudy or visually unappealing. In fact, many people remove and discard this substance, incorrectly believing it is unhealthy or contamination within the bottle. But in fact, they are removing the most healthy, beneficial portion of the vinegar.

Mother of vinegar is a rich source of iron, which not only naturally enables the body to create essential hemoglobin used to oxygenate the blood, but also aids in proper functioning of the body. It is also an excellent source of vitamin B, plus is high in prebiotics which can help balance good and bad bacteria within the body.

Mother is most commonly found in home made vinegar where intensive curing and filtering rarely takes place. It can also be present in store bought varieties, but this is mostly limited to the unpasteurized types. In fact, most commercially manufactured vinegar intentionally filters out mother and any other visible "imperfections" as the general public tends to misunderstand this as being visually unattractive and less desirable. In reality, this extraction is not only harmless, but would be removing the most beneficial part of the vinegar.

This jelly-like substance is proven to be full of concentrated nutrients essential to good health. It is believed to aid in the fighting of bacterial infections, digestion and weight loss, in addition to treating a nearly endless list of adverse health conditions.

While mother of vinegar can be eaten, it is best to consume a serving of the unpurified vinegar which is benefitting from the substance. Consider this a type of probiotic solution that is gaining so much momentum in natural health circles today. This unfiltered solution can be taken daily as a preventative for better digestive health, to build a stronger immune system, as well as a host of additional benefits. Probiotics such as this, serve as food for good bacteria in the body's intestines. Strengthening this portion of the digestive tract aids in overall digestion, and prevents issues associated with a sick bowel.

In addition to consuming mother, the thick gel can also be strained out and used to cultivate a brand new batch of high quality vinegar.

The attributes and composition of vinegar have been well documented by numerous researchers through the last several decades. This leads us to the most pertinent aspect of vinegar — how we can directly benefit from its use! The chapters that follow give you tangible ways vinegar can be used to positively impact your life for better health and vigorous living!

Chapter Two
Vinegar Home Remedies

Research studies indicate what people throughout the world have known for generations — vinegar, particularly the apple cider type, contains the means to not only promote better health, but also prevent and cure disease. Studies link vinegar to a stronger immune system, as well as fighting an astounding number of ailments and condition.

The use of vinegar in home remedies can be noted throughout recorded history. It was prevalent in Biblical accounts, and considered a treasured asset in Cleopatra's time. History records vinegar being used to treat wounded soldiers on the battlefield dating as far back as war itself, all the way through the United States' bloody Civil War and beyond.

One of the most fabled accounts of medicinal vinegar came during the black plague of medieval times. As villages were being ravaged by the deadly disease, four plundering thieves cheated death by wrapping their faces with vinegar and herbed soaked cloths as they looted their way across infected towns. Whether this was fact or fiction may never be truly known, but it does represent the belief many hold extolling vinegar's potent use as a natural healing agent.

Vinegar's place in medicinal circles

It is a well known fact that Hippocrates himself, the "father" of modern medicine, relied on vinegar as a treatment for the sick and infirmed. In fact, today's medicinal field has also recognized and adopted vinegar as both a treatment and preventative for numerous medical conditions — even replacing available pharmaceutical options in its favor.

Vinegar's natural composition makes it a potent bacterial and viral fighter without the harmful side effects and addictive qualities prevalent in so many modern day medicines. It is all-natural, and works in conjunction with the body's own chemistry to fight disease. Not only does vinegar combat infection, but also helps restore depleted minerals and nutrients in throughout the body for better overall health.

Physicians' offices and hospitals throughout the world have begun to use some of the same home remedy vinegar methods on their patients that our great grandparents passed down for generations. Medical facilities depend on vinegar for everything from treating bacterial ear infections to cleaning and disinfecting medical equipment from contamination. And scientific research studies are on-going in the determination of additional ways vinegar can be beneficial to patients on a variety of levels.

Giving Vinegar a Try

The following pages introduce you to the world of vinegar as a natural home health remedy. Give these tips a try, remembering that some are tried and true methods handed down for generations, while others are being used throughout medical facilities worldwide. Some still may have been rooted in folklore, but only you can decide which remedies work best for you. Every body carries its own distinct characteristics, and reacts differently to outside stimuli. What may work wonders for a friend's arthritis, for example, may seem ineffective to you. Likewise, your newly found treatment for gout may bring you new found relief, but still be lacking for others. Bottom line, don't be afraid to try new relief methods until you find which remedy (or remedies) is the right fit for you. Relief is out there...it is up to you to continue searching until you find it.

And before beginning any new health regimen, even one that is natural and homeopathic in nature, it is always best to consult your healthcare provider. Be certain to provide him or her with a list of current medications you are taking, along with the natural course of action you would like to try. After all, we are all working together in this quest for better living!

Enjoy!

The "Original" Daily Vinegar Tonic

The very best way to combat disease is through prevention before illness sets in. Looking for an easy way to incorporate vinegar into your daily routine for better health and wellness? Sometimes the best way is the most simple way. Try drinking 1 teaspoon of apple cider vinegar first thing in the morning for a stronger immune system and disease prevention.

Using Vinegar to Prevent Illness

Daily Vinegar Tonics

Vinegar tonics can be used daily as not only a preventative for disease, but also to help build the body's immune system. Combine 1 tablespoon apple cider vinegar in an 8 ounce glass of water and drink daily for better wellness.

Another Daily Vinegar Tonic

Some people swear by the power of a daily bout of apple cider vinegar to improve their health. But the tonic only works if it is palatable enough to consume on a daily basis! For better tasting vinegar, try mixing 1 teaspoon of honey with the tablespoon of apple cider vinegar in your 8 ounce glass of water. This tonic can be consumed two to three times a day, if desired.

More Daily Vinegar Tonics

If the robust flavor of vinegar is too much for you, or if you are just looking for something a little different from time to time, there is nothing wrong with mixing things up and experimenting a little! For example, a teaspoon or two of vinegar can be added to a small glass of fruit juice or most of your favorite beverages — even warm tea. In many cases, you may not even notice the addition of vinegar to the taste of your drink, but will still reap all its health benefits! Don't be afraid to play around with different flavor combinations until you find one that best suits your personal taste.

Before Dinner Vinegar Tonic

The benefits of taking in a glass of vinegar tonic before dinner are two fold. First, you can count on benefitting from all the wonderful health attributes associated with vinegar. But second, drinking apple cider vinegar before a meal may help aid in the digestive process. Its potent enzymes not only help digestion, but are also known to prevent gas and bloating.

Vinegar Detox

For a detoxifying effect, try combining 2 tablespoons of apple cider vinegar, 1 tablespoon of lemon juice, 1 teaspoon of honey, 1/4 teaspoon of ginger in an 8 ounce glass of warm water. Local, raw honey always works best, as this helps provide a natural immunity against various allergies.

Natural Home Remedies

Acid Reflux

To combat the symptoms of acid reflux, combine 1 teaspoon of apple cider vinegar into a cup of water and drink. Vinegar can work as a natural balance to pH levels in the body's digestive system to help neutralize stomach acid.

Allergies

Combine 1 tablespoon apple cider vinegar with 2 teaspoons of raw honey in a cup of water. Drink this mixture twice a day to head off seasonal allergies. It is important to use local honey, if at all possible. Using local honey can help reduce allergy symptoms and even build up the body's natural immunity to local pollens and fauna that trigger seasonal allergies.

Arthritis

The pain of arthritis can prove debilitating and interfere with every aspect of daily life. Anti-inflammatory properties widely associated with apple cider vinegar make it a potent choice for relief from arthritis pain. Combine 1 teaspoon of apple cider vinegar in a glass of warm water. Stir in a teaspoon of honey and sip on it like a tea. For most promising results, drink one glass in the morning and a second in the evening before bedtime.

Stronger Arthritis Relief

Several ingredients in this arthritis concoction have properties conducive to relief from arthritis pain. In addition to the already discussed anti-inflammatory properties found in apple cider vinegar, celery contains luteolin which also claims the same benefit. Grapefruit is another ingredient rich in inflammation-fighting antioxidants. Together, these make for a powerful choice in pain relief.

Leaving the peelings on the fruit, cut 2 stalks of celery, 1 orange, 1/2 grapefruit and lemon into chunks, and simmer in 4 cups of water for an hour, or until they become tender. Press the softened foods through a tight sieve, into a bowl. Add in 1 tablespoon apple cider vinegar and about a tablespoon of salt.

When ready, combine 1/4 cup of this mixture into a full glass of water, drinking one glass in the morning, and the second in the evening.

Arthritis Relief Tonic

Prevention is the best medicine. This simple tonic can be used to head off bouts of arthritis *before* they occur. Combine 2 teaspoons of apple cider vinegar into a cup of water. Drink this mixture before each meal, three times a day to keep swelling down and stave off arthritis.

Arthritis Pain Relief

During an arthritis flare up, pain relief can be hard to come by. Try this combination when arthritis pain needs addressed. Mix 1 cup of apple cider vinegar, 1/2 cup local honey, 1/2 cup blueberries, 1/2 cup raspberries and 1 teaspoon lemon juice in a blender. Combine until blueberries have popped and everything is thoroughly mixed. Take 2 or 3 tablespoons each day for pain relief.

Arthritis Poultice (do not ingest)

Apple cider vinegar contains a storehouse of nutrients and minerals that can help ease arthritis pain. It is naturally high in calcium and magnesium, which help keep joints in optimal working condition. Its antioxidants mend damaged tissue, and the alkaline in vinegar reduces swelling and inflammation, making it a potent fighter against arthritis when taken daily. But what many people don't realize is that vinegar can also work outside the body to reduce the pain and swelling of arthritis.

To make your own poultice wrap, combine 1/2 cup apple cider vinegar, 2 egg whites, 1/2 cup of turpentine and 1/4 cup olive oil in a small disposable tub. Using a soft cloth, massage this mixture into aching joints for relief from pain. DO NOT INGEST. If desired, you can also try excluding the turpentine from this recipe.

Arthritis Wrap

Try this arthritis wrap on aching joints. Combine 1 and 1/2 cups of apple cider vinegar with 3 cups of very warm (not hot) water. Soak a soft cloth in the mixture and wrap warm, soaked cloth around joint for relief.

Arthritis Soak

Pour 2 cups of apple cider vinegar into a bathtub of warm water. Carefully climb into tub and soak aching joints while the water is warm. Works best if you can stay in the water for 20 to 30 minutes.

Arthritis Rub

Combine 1 tablespoon of vinegar with 2 teaspoons of olive oil and gently warm. Rub this combination into an aching joint for relief. Keep a supply of this on hand and use several times throughout the day during more frequent bouts of arthritis.

Athlete's Foot

Athlete's foot is a type of fungus, which makes vinegar's antifungal properties a great match for treating this type of irritation. One of the simplest treatments for athlete's foot is to soak your feet for 20 to 30 minutes in a pan or small bucket filled with apple cider vinegar. If you do not have apple cider vinegar, distilled (white) vinegar can also be used. After soaking, be sure to gently dry off your feet. It is always important for feet infected with athlete's foot to stay dry.

Athlete's Foot Spot Treatment

At the first sign of athlete's foot, or for smaller, spotty infections, just dab a bit of undiluted apple cider vinegar onto a soft cloth or cotton ball. Use this to directly treat the affected areas several times a day until gone.

Athlete's Foot Treatment and Prevention

One of the best ways to prevent athlete's foot and to keep it from spreading is to thoroughly clean and disinfect socks and stockings. In a large bowl or small bucket, combine 1 cup of apple cider vinegar with about 5 cups of water. Place socks and stockings in this solution and allow to soak for about 30 minutes. Then, wash and dry as usual.

Asthma

For those suffering from asthma, prevention is the best policy. Apple cider vinegar may help ward off many asthma encounters, simply by helping to stave off attacks in the first place.

Try a cup of prevention. In your favorite teacup, fill with warm water, 1 tablespoon apple cider vinegar and a teaspoon or so of honey. Stir together and drink in the morning before an asthma episode even begins. To make this more a part of your everyday routine, the apple cider vinegar and honey can even be added to your favorite morningtime tea for a more flavorful and palatable approach.

Asthma Episodes

Studies by the Cleveland Clinic Foundation indicate that up to 75% of asthma sufferers also deal with some type of gastroesophageal reflux disease (or GERD), and that this reflux may contribute to difficulty in breathing in asthma patients. As the esophagus constricts or narrows due to reflux, these patients can find themselves struggling to breathe. The acidity associated with apple cider vinegar may be helpful in reducing reflux, therefore relieving the constriction.

Try sipping on 1 tablespoon of apple cider vinegar mixed into a glass of warm water over the course of about 45 minutes. You do not need to ingest the total amount all at once. Little sips spread out over a short amount of time may slowly work to open the esophagus and relieve symptoms.

Asthma Acupressure Trick

Acupressure has also been known to relieve asthmatic symptoms. Simply soak a gauze pad in apple cider vinegar, and rid of any dripping excess. Pad should still remain as wet as possible without dripping. Use rubber bands to hold the soaked gauze pad in place on the inside of the wrists for relief. Be sure the rubber bands are snug enough to hold the pad in place, but not tight enough to interfere with circulation or become irritating.

Backaches

Treat an aching back with a warm apple cider vinegar soak. Fill a bathtub full of warm water and add 2 cups of apple cider vinegar. Soak with your back in the water for 20 to 30 minutes for relief.

Backache Compress

Soak a soft cloth or small, light towel in a solution of 1 cup very warm water and 1 cup apple cider vinegar. Wring out excess solution, but keep moistened towel as wet as possible. Lay on stomach and drape warm vinegar towel across aching back. Allow compress to stay in place while warm, for 10 to 20 minutes. Repeat as needed.

Bladder Infection

Vinegar's antiseptic qualities make it a potent choice for the relief of bladder infections. Simply combine 1 tablespoon apple cider vinegar in a cup of water and drink 2 or 3 times a day to end the infection.

Bladder Infection Juice

Another simple way to help flush out a bladder infection is by ramping up everyday cranberry juice. Cranberry juice is a well-known go-to remedy for bladder infections, and has been passed down in health circles for generation with great success. To increase the potency of the cranberry juice solution, try adding a tablespoon of apple cider vinegar to your glass of cranberry juice.

Boils

Painful boils can be treated with a solution of vinegar and willow. Simmer together 1 cup of apple cider vinegar and 1/4 cup fresh, broken willow twigs. Continue simmering until twigs are tender and bendable. Drench this warm (not hot) liquid into a soft cloth and use as a poultice on tender, painful skin boils.

Try to avoid popping the boil, but instead resoak with a warm vinegar compress and allow this action to bring any puss or discharge to the top of the boil on its own. If boil should break, be sure to keep the area clean and dry to avoid infection.

Calluses

To rid hands and feet of calluses, dip half a slice of stale bread directly into apple cider vinegar, and secure into place on top of calluses before bed. Remove in the morning and repeat until calluses soften.

Callus Thickening

More difficult and thickened calluses may benefit from apple cider vinegar's high acid content. This acid is great at breaking up and reducing hardened areas of the skin. Combine 1/2 cup vinegar with 2 cups of warm water and soak callused area for about 20 minutes, several times a day. Be sure and dry area thoroughly after treatment.

More Calluses

For a more direct approach to eliminating calluses, try soaking a cotton ball in undiluted apple cider vinegar. Use a piece of medical tape to fasten the cotton ball on the affected area for about 30 minutes to see if this helps soften the callus. Repeat, if needed, being careful not to tear the skin.

Cholesterol

The idea behind using apple cider vinegar to reduce cholesterol is understanding that pectin, found abundantly in all varieties of apples, slows the body's absorption of food in the intestinal tract. As this process has been slowed, LDL (bad cholesterol) now has time to attach itself to the pectin found abundantly in vinegar and is removed. Using apple cider vinegar to reduce cholesterol is particularly helpful if the body's cholesterol levels are elevated due to a poor diet. Vinegar may be able to offset this.

Two or three tablespoons of apple cider vinegar added to your favorite drink, such as juice or even sparkling water, can be beneficial in lowering this type of cholesterol over time.

Cholesterol Concoction

In addition to using apple cider vinegar, this combination of ingredients brings in the medicinal effects of both cinnamon and honey for a more potent formula. In a blender, add 1 cup apple cider vinegar, 2 cups chopped apples (any kind), 1/2 cup honey, and 1/2 teaspoon of both cinnamon and nutmeg. Blend together until well combined. Sip a few teaspoons of this fortified vinegar throughout the day to gradually help lower cholesterol.

Colds

Try dealing with the common cold with this old-time remedy that has been passed down for generations. Soak an 8" square of brown paper (from a paper grocery bag) in apple cider vinegar. Sprinkle one side of the wet brown paper with cayenne pepper and lay it directly onto the chest, keeping it in place for 15 to 20 minutes. Remove the used paper and wash the chest clean, taking care not to become chilled.

Congestion

Apple cider vinegar has long been used to combat common

congestion. One of the most effective uses is to add about 1/4 cup of vinegar to vaporizer water and allow the vinegar vapors to penetrate the air. Breathing in this steam will help break up mucus and ease congestion, allowing for easier breathing.

More Congestion

Using a couple of soft, clean cloths, soak them in undiluted apple cider vinegar and wrap around wrists at bedtime to help ease congestion and breathe better throughout the night, when congestion tends to become worse.

Congestion Tonic

Try this simple tonic to relieve congestion. A small batch can be made in the morning and sipped throughout the day. Combine 1 cup apple cider vinegar with 1 to 2 tablespoons of honey, 1 clove of minced garlic and a pinch of cayenne pepper. Great for relieving deep congestion.

Constipation

Pectin, found in abundance in apple cider vinegar, is a water-soluble fiber that researchers believe can help promote better digestion and eliminate constipation. For a simple go-to remedy, combine 2 tablespoon vinegar and 1 teaspoon of lemon juice into a cup of water. Try this combination 3 times a day to end constipation.

Constipation Elixir

Adding apple cider vinegar to already pectin-heavy apple juice can be a great way to end constipation. Just mix 2 tablespoons of vinegar into your favorite brand of apple juice and enjoy!

More Congestion

Using a couple of soft, clean cloths, soak them in undiluted apple cider vinegar and wrap gently around wrists at bedtime. This will help ease congestion and allow for easier breathing throughout the night, when congestion tends to become worse.

Corns

Ridding yourself of painful corns can be easy using this two-step approach. First, fill a bucket with very warm (not hot) soapy water and add 1 to 1/2 cups apple cider vinegar. Soak foot in warm water solution for about 20 minutes as corns begin to soften. After soaking feet, apply a dab or two of olive oil to the corn and allow to penetrate. After a few minutes, place socks on feet to eliminate any chance of slipping, or go directly to bed with oil on feet and allow to soak overnight.

Cough

To end a nagging cough, combine 1/4 cup apple cider vinegar with 2 tablespoons of honey into a drinking glass of water. Drink this solution once in the morning and once in the evening before bedtime.

Cough Syrup

Make your own completely natural cough syrup from two of herbalists favorite ingredients: apple cider vinegar and honey. Combine 1/2 cup apple cider vinegar with 2 tablespoons of honey. This solution works best when slightly warmed and sipped throughout the day to end a nagging cough. 1 clove of minced garlic can also be added to the solution for an even stronger kick.

Stronger Cough Syrup

Making your own cough syrup is both simple and beneficial. Simple, because the ingredients are probably already in your kitchen pantry, and beneficial because you can make it as strong or as palatable as you like. Begin with 1/4 cup apple cider vinegar and add 1/4 cup honey, 1 clove minced garlic, 1/2 teaspoon ground cinnamon and 1/8 teaspoon cayenne pepper in a glass jar. Combine well and sip a bit throughout the day to relieve your cough. Not only are you getting the well-known health benefits and cough suppressant qualities in apple cider vinegar, but the same attributes associated with the additional herbs as well. If the mixture is too strong (or weak) for your liking, simply adjust the amounts of the added herbs to your liking.

Pillowcase Cough Solution

Using undiluted apple cider vinegar, sprinkle a clean pillowcase with the vinegar just before bedtime to soothe a dry, nightime cough. Gently inhaling the aroma will help to sooth a cough and keep air passageways open for a more restful sleep.

Diabetes

Research from the Arizona State University is one of several studies that suggest apple cider vinegar may help control type 2 diabetes by reducing glucose levels when consumed before meals. Combine 2 tablespoons of apple cider vinegar with 1/8 teaspoon of salt in a glass (8 ounce) of water. Drink before lunch and dinner meals to help reduce glucose levels.

Diabetes Control

Some studies have shown that something as simple as adding a few teaspoonfuls of apple cider vinegar to your meal can significantly reduce glucose spikes in patients with type 2 diabetes. Using vinegar to help bring down glucose counts in diabetics doesn't have to be complicated. It's as easy as including apple cider vinegar in your meal planning. What simpler way to accomplish this than the addition of apple cider vinegar as a dressing over salad greens or as an accompaniment to a side of vegetables.

Diabetic Control Before Bedtime

Interesting research has also shown that the combination of a simple snack of apple cider vinegar and cheese right before bedtime can also help bring down glucose levels in diabetics. Next time you are looking for a delicious, yet healthy, snack before sleep, why not try this vinegar and cheese solution?

Simple Solution to Diabetes Control Before Meals

For diabetics who also need to curb their sodium intake, try combining 2 tablespoons of apple cider vinegar into a glass (8 ounces) of water and consuming before mealtime. You will not be burdened with the added sodium some remedies contain, but still receive the benefits of more stabilized blood sugar levels.

Diabetes and Hypoglycemia

A research study by the *Journal of Diabetes Research* reveals that vinegar can help reduce hypoglycemia in type 2 diabetes patients. Why not try adding just a tablespoon or two of apple cider vinegar to your favorite dinnertime beverage, such as iced tea? Many people claim to reap the health benefits of the vinegar addition, but do not notice much difference in taste when combined with another beverage.

Diarrhea

Vinegar has long been used throughout history to help end bouts of diarrhea. Its antibiotic properties help in killing off parasitic and bacterial organisms that may be causing the diarrhea bout in the first place. Loaded with pectin, it can also help to sooth and settle an irritated colon. For best results, mix 1 teaspoon apple cider vinegar into a cup of water and drink 2 to 4 times throughout the day.

Diarrhea Dehydration

Because apple cider vinegar helps balance pH levels in the gut and digestive tract, it can also be beneficial for not only alleviating diarrhea, but also supplementing essential minerals and nutrients which can be lost with accompanying dehydration. Combine 2 tablespoons apple cider vinegar with 1 teaspoon of honey in a cup of water. Drink this solution 3 or 4 times daily until diarrhea subsides.

Ear Infections

Homeopathic circles have long depended on vinegar to treat ear infections. But science has shown this is no longer considered fringe or folklore. Ohio State University's hospital routinely prescribes vinegar irrigation treatment for chronic middle ear infections. One of the simplest ways to administer a vinegar treatment to the ear follows.

Tilt the head toward your shoulder allowing your ear to face the ceiling. Pour a teaspoonful of white (distilled) vinegar directly into the ear canal, making certain the solution flows all the way down into the canal (covering any infection). Keep vinegar in the ear for about 30 seconds, and then tip your ear upright again to drain the vinegar solution onto a paper towel. Repeat three times a day until ear infection has cleared up.

Swimmers Ear

Swimmers is a sometimes painful bacterial or fungal infection located in the outer portion of the ear canal. It is caused by moisture being trapped in the ear canal after bathing or swimming. Swimmers ear can be treated with a few doses of white (distilled) vinegar being poured down the ear canal and allowed to set for a few minutes before draining. Many people also use a warm heating pad on the ear to help ease pain until fully cleared up.

Swimmers Ear Prevention

Additional research has been conducted by the American Academy of Otolaryngology into the use of vinegar as a treatment to prevent and treat swimmer's ear infections. Use this method after swimming in a pond or lake to prevent water-borne infections from settling into the ear. Combine 3 tablespoons distilled vinegar and 3 tablespoons rubbing alcohol in a small dish. Using an eye dropper (and without putting the dropper into the actual ear), gently rinse and irrigate the ear canal to eliminate any bacteria which may work to form an infection later.

Eczema

Apple cider vinegar contains a storehouse of properties that make it ideal for treating skin ailments such as eczema. It is both antifungal and antibacterial which helps its effectiveness in maintaining healthy skin. Not only can it help rid skin of eczema, it also balances delicate pH levels leaving skin blemish-free and glowing.

Using a soft cloth soaked in undiluted apple cider vinegar, gently dab onto areas of skin effected with eczema and allow to air dry. Try this twice a day until dissipated.

Eczema from the Inside Out

Combine 2 teaspoons of apple cider vinegar with 1 teaspoon of honey is a glass (8 ounces) of water. Drink this blend 2 or 3 times a day for one week to eliminate eczema and hydrate the skin.

Electrolytes

Heat, exercise and illness can all cause the body to become depleted of essential electrolytes. To restore these necessary elements, mix 1 tablespoon of apple cider vinegar into a glass of water and consume after exercising or working in the hot afternoon sun. It is also a wonderful solution to restore these elements during bouts of illness.

Fatigue

For rapid relief with bouts of fatigue, combine 1 teaspoon apple cider vinegar with 1 teaspoon of honey into a glass of water. Drink the entire cup to become re-energized and refreshed.

Food Poisoning Prevention

Some physicians recommend consuming vinegar whenever eating questionable food sources, such as what can oftentimes happen when traveling to a foreign country. This remedy can and should be used for the entire travel period as a preventative measure. Simply add 1 tablespoon of apple cider vinegar to another drinking beverage. Local stream or tap water should always be avoided. Oftentimes, these water sources may be the problem). Drink the apple cider vinegar addition as a preventative measure 30 minutes before meals. If the taste of vinegar becomes too strong, a dollop of honey can be added to make it more palatable.

Foot Aches

Aching feet can be effectively treated with a warm vinegar bath application. Simply add about 3/4 cup of apple cider vinegar to a bathtub filled about 6 inches deep with warm water. Walk back and forth in the water, taking care not to slip. Try this first thing in the morning for about 5 minutes, and then again in the evening before bed for an additional 5 minutes.

For people with balance issues where falling may be a concern, you can use this same idea to sit on the edge of the bathtub with your feet soaking in the water. Just be sure to sway your feet around the water as much as possible, even massaging the warm vinegar water into joints and the ankle area while soaking. Press and massage the balls of the feet for added comfort and relief. Try this method 2 or 3 times daily, as needed.

In both cases, be certain to thoroughly dry feet when you are finished to avoid slipping on the bathroom floor.

Foot Ache Wrap

For particularly aching feet, thoroughly soak a soft cloth or towel in a warm apple cider vinegar and water solution. Try a 50-50 combination for this. Wring out any excess liquid just so the cloth isn't dripping and wrap snugly around feet. Allow this wrap to remain in place while warm, even massaging the foot while it is being wrapped. When the cloth loses its warm, remove it and be sure to dry your feet completely before walking to avoid slippage. Repeat several times throughout the day, as necessary.

Gas

Gas can be not only a nuisance, but is oftentimes painful. Apple cider vinegar can help alleviate uncomfortable gas pains quickly and easily. Just mix 1 teaspoonful of apple cider vinegar into a glass of warm water and drink slowly. The natural healing elements found so abundantly in vinegar will work swiftly to neutralize many causes of gas in the digestive tract.

Gas Preventative

To prevent troublesome gas beforehand, try sipping on a teaspoonful of apple cider vinegar in a glass of water or your favorite tea right before eating dinner. This will help head off many of the dietary causes of gas, from certain vegetables for example, before it becomes a problem.

Headaches

Headaches are caused by numerous reasons: some stress-oriented, others more medical in nature. Regardless of the cause, when headaches hit, relief needs to come swiftly. Apple cider vinegar can be a priceless remedy for bouts of headaches. The key is finding which remedy works best for you personally, do bring relief quickly and effectively. That may mean trying several remedies before stumbling on the one that's best suited for the source of your headache in conjunction with your body's own chemistry.

For starters, combine 1 cup of apple cider vinegar with 1 cup of water on the stove and bring to a boil. Carefully pour the heated water into a large bowl and place on the table. Cover your head with a towel over the bowl, and allow vapors to rise. Breathe in these warm, aromatic vapors for 5 to 10 minutes to bring relief from headaches.

Headache Relief

Combine 1/4 cup apple cider vinegar with 1/4 cup warm water. Soak a clean cloth in the solution and wring out any excess moisture so that fabric is not dripping wet. Place wet cloth across forehead and temple area. Lay in a quiet, dark room for 20 minutes to bring relief from a headache.

Headache Vaporizer

Using an old-fashioned vaporizer can still be one of the most effective means of ending a nagging headache. Add about 1/4 cup of apple cider vinegar to the water in your vaporizer, and inhale for 5 minutes. This remedy works best by laying in a dark, quiet room for at least 30 minutes following treatment.

And always make sure that vaporizers are left clean after using, to avoid bacterial germ build up that can make people ill.

Headaches and Brown Paper Bags

Another old-time remedy that still works can be found in this brown paper bag treatment. Using a grocery story-type paper bag, soak the bottom of the open edges in a basin of undiluted apple cider vinegar. Put the bag on your head, much like you would a chef's hat, and tie it in place with a long scarf. Sit quietly and gently inhale the fumes. Your headache should be relieved in about 45 minutes.

Headaches Caused by Elevated Blood Pressure

Elevated blood pressure and headaches go hand in hand. For these types of headaches, try this remedy that is specially formulated.

Celery is naturally high is magnesium, potassium and fiber —
all things known to help stabilize high blood pressure. Using
celery in conjunction with the nutritional elements already found
abundantly in apple cider vinegar and you have a powerful blood
pressure reducer.

Cut 2 celery stalks in half and boil them in 2 cups of apple cider
vinegar. Remove the pan from heat and allow to cool completely.
At first sign of a headache caused by raised blood pressure, chew
on a vinegar-fortified celery stalk for relief.

Heartburn

At the first sign of heartburn, sip on a little swig of undiluted apple
cider vinegar to neutralize acid and balance stomach pH levels.

Heartburn Tonic

To reverse the acidity in the stomach associated with heartburn,
drink a tall glass of water to which 1 teaspoon of apple cider
vinegar has been added. This can be done either prior to a meal, or
during the meal itself.

Heartburn Prevention

For quick relief from heartburn, add 2 teaspoons of apple cider
vinegar into about 3/4 cup of water. Drink 10 minutes prior to
eating a meal to prevent heartburn.

Hiccups

To bring an end to a bout of irritating hiccups, mix 1 teaspoon of
apple cider vinegar into a cup of warm water. Sip on this solution
very slowly to rid yourself of hiccups.

High Blood Pressure

Researchers are beginning to study the positive effects vinegar
has on lowering high blood pressure. Some studies show that

consuming just a teaspoonful of apple cider vinegar each day may help bring blood pressure down and keep it down.

Hives

Vinegar contains wonderful antiseptic properties that make it the perfect natural health remedy for treating itchy hives. Combine 1 tablespoon of apple cider vinegar with 1 tablespoon of cornstarch, forming it into a thick paste. Use this paste to blot onto itchy areas of the skin and allow to completely dry. Gently wash off paste with warm water, followed by a cool rinse. Repeat as often as necessary to bring relief.

Indigestion

Many of the body's digestive issues can benefit from apple cider vinegar. Vinegar is a natural pH balancer in addition to being an overall aid to the digestive tract. As such, you will see it is recommended from a multitude of sources. A basic remedy for indigestion is to combine 1 cup of apple cider vinegar in a jar with 2 teaspoons of honey and a teaspoon of freshly grated ginger root. Use this to sip after a meal that has left you with indigestion.

Influenza

Vinegar has long been used as a cleaning agent to disinfect areas of the house contaminated with the flu virus. It contains natural antibacterial and antiviral properties that make it a potent weapon against influenza outbreaks.

Bring 2 to 4 cups of apple cider vinegar to a boil over medium heat. Continue to boil the vinegar, uncovered, allowing the vapors to permeate the entire room. After the vinegar has been reduced by about half, use the remaining vinegar to wipe down countertops, door knobs and anywhere else viral germs can accumulate.

Insect Bites and Stings

To take the "sting" out of insect bites, soak a cotton ball in apple cider vinegar and gently dab over bug bites and stings to relieve pain and itching.

Insect Bites Healing Paste

Form a thick paste to place on the top of itchy insect bites by combining 1 tablespoon of apple cider vinegar with 1 tablespoon of baking soda. After the initial foaming action takes place, continue to combine until a paste forms, adding more baking soda or vinegar until it reaches the consistency of toothpaste. Use this blend to place onto aggravated areas and allow to dry completely. Then, wash off with warm water and follow with a cool water rinse. Pat dry and repeat as often as necessary for relief.

Insomnia

Dealing with a lack of sleep can produce all sorts of negative effects on the body. Insomnia has not only been linked to illness by lowering the body's immune system, but also impairs cognitive function and can increase depression. Ensuring a good night's rest is essential to better living.

To help combat depression, combine 1 tablespoon of apple cider vinegar with 3/4 cup of honey and set aside for bedtime. About 20 minutes prior to going to bed, consume 1 teaspoon of this mixture, saving the remainder for the next evening.

Remember the key to getting a good night's rest lays in keeping your body in a routine. Begin establishing a good bedtime routine, incorporating the teaspoon of the apple cider and honey mixture, and sticking to it. As your body gets more accustomed to the routine, you will find yourself getting better and better rest each night.

Insulin Spikes

Scientific research studies have shown that apple cider vinegar can reduce insulin and glucose levels in the bloodstream. If insulin spikes are a concern, consume 1 teaspoonful of apple cider vinegar immediately prior to mealtime to keep levels in check.

Leg Cramps

For relief of leg cramping, try this long-time home remedy. Combine 1 teaspoon of apple cider vinegar and an equal teaspoon of honey with 1 tablespoon of calcium lactate. Mix this into 3/4 cup of warm water and stir until completely dissolved and combined. Drink this entire solution once daily to prevent nighttime leg cramps.

Leg Cramp Prevention

Get into the habit of drinking a simple glass of water in which 1 tablespoon of apple cider vinegar has been added with meals to prevent leg cramps.

Muscle Aches

To relieve the body of aching muscles, pour 2 cups of apple cider vinegar into a bath of warm (not hot) water. Soak in the warm tub for at least 20 minutes each day to heal a sore body.

Muscle Aches (poultice)

Make your own poultice for healing aching muscles. Combine 1/4 cup apple cider vinegar with 2 wintergreen sprigs. Soak a clean cloth in the vinegar solution, and apply to sore muscles for 10 minutes at a time. Repeat as often as needed.

Muscle Aches (additional poultice)

Combine 1/2 cup of apple cider vinegar and 1/4 teaspoon of cayenne pepper in a dish. Soak a soft, clean cloth in the vinegar solution and wring out any dripping moisture, still keeping the cloth wet. Apple to sore muscles and keep in place for at least 5 minutes, 3 times a day.

Muscle Aches (penetrating poultice)

Gently warm (but do not boil) 1 or 2 cups of undiluted apple cider vinegar on the stove top. While still warm, but cool enough to handle without getting burned, soak a clean, soft cloth in vinegar until saturated. Wring out excess moisture and wrap around aching muscle to enjoy deep, penetrating muscle relief for 10 to 15 minutes at a time. You can repeat this method throughout the day as needed.

Nasal Congestion

For relief of nasal congestion, try this home remedy. Combine 1 cup of apple cider vinegar with 1 cup of water in a small saucepan. Bring to a boil on the stovetop. Once boiling, carefully pour solution into a wide bowl and place on the tabletop. Cover your head with a towel over the bowl, and breathe in vapors allowing them to help reduce congestion.

Nausea

To combat bouts of nausea, combine 1 tablespoon of apple cider vinegar and 1 tablespoon of honey in 1 1/2 cups of water. Slowly sip on the mixture to bring relief from an upset stomach. You may also benefit from making a small batch of this concoction to have it readily on hand for nausea relief.

Nausea Solution

Try this easy solution to end nausea. Combine 2 teaspoons of apple cider vinegar with 2 teaspoons of raw, local honey. At the first sign of nausea, consume the entire amount.

Nausea (poultice)

Apple cider vinegar can be useful for fighting nausea both inside the body as well as outside. Consider using this helpful poultice when episodes of nausea arrive.

Gently warm 1/4 cup of apple cider vinegar over the stove. Soak a soft, clean cloth in the vinegar allowing it to soak up all the liquid. Wring out any excess moisture, but still leave the cloth plenty wet. Lay down and place the warm vinegar cloth directly on your stomach. As the cloth cools, replace with a newly warmed poultice as needed until nausea subsides.

Nosebleeds
To effectively stop a nosebleed, use this old cure. Saturate a cotton ball in apple cider vinegar and gently squeeze out the excess. Place wet cotton ball in nostril with the bleed. Nosebleed will stop as the vinegar helps the blood to congeal.

Nosebleeds (preventative)
The use of a vinegar drink can help prevent nosebleeds in the first place. Drink a daily combination of 2 teaspoons of apple cider vinegar with 3/4 cup of water to help prevent bleeds.

PMS Cramping
Some women have found relief from premenstrual cramping by drinking a solution of 2 teaspoons of apple cider vinegar mixed into a warm glass of water.

PMS Symptoms
Premenstrual symptoms run the gamut, and are different for each woman. Vinegar not only contains minerals and nutrients essential for proper body function, but can also help balance hormone levels. Simply mix 1 teaspoon of apple cider vinegar into a cup of water and drink twice daily for relief of PMS symptoms.

Pneumonia

Help ease the pneumonic chest by pouring 2 cups of apple cider vinegar into a small pan and bringing to a boil over medium heat. Continue to boil the vinegar uncovered, allowing the vapors to flow throughout the room, gently breathing them in.

Shingles

The pain of shingles can be both deep and lasting. And, many of the over-the-counter treatments to control pain fall short. Get back to basics by using this natural remedy for relief.

Combine 3 tablespoons of apple cider vinegar with 3 tablespoons of cornstarch, forming a thick paste. Once mixed, use this paste to gently coat painful shingle lesions by carefully dabbing it onto the skin and allowing it to dry completely. When needed, gently rinse dried paste away with cool water and pat dry with a soft, clean cloth. This paste can be applied as often as needed for quick, cooling relief, so be sure and keep extra on hand.

Shingles (more)

Using a soft cloth, saturate with apple cider vinegar and wring out the majority of the moisture, just enough that the wet cloth is not dripping. Place saturated cloth directly over shingle lesions for cool relief. Once used, be sure to wash the cloth in hot, sanitizing water to clean completely as to not spread the disease.

Skin Infections

This remedy works for a variety of different skin ailments. For infections of the skin, soak a clean, dry cloth in undiluted apple cider vinegar and wring out the extra moisture. Place the vinegar-soaked cloth directly on the infected area of the skin to heal long lasting and stubborn infections. Vinegar's germ-fighting ability can help eliminate bacteria on the skin and speed up the healing of infection.

Sore Throat

This well-known sore throat tonic has been passed down from generation to generation with good reason. It is both potent and effective.

Combine 1/4 cup of apple cider vinegar with 1/4 cup raw, local honey. Set aside for use as needed. When a sore throat hits, consume 1 tablespoon of this mixture every 4 hours for relief. It also may be taken more often, if necessary.

Sore Throat Gargle

Combine 1 tablespoon of white (distilled) vinegar with a cup of water. Use this to gargle away a throat infection 2 or 3 times a day for effective relief.

Sore Throat Tonic

Combine this tonic and keep near the bedside during an illness with a nagging sore throat.

Mix 1/2 cup of apple cider vinegar, 1/2 cup of water, 1 teaspoon cayenne pepper and 3 tablespoons of honey. Use this to gently sip on for relief.

Sprains

For muscle sprains that require a hot soak, fill a clean bucket with hot water (but not scalding). Add a cup of apple cider vinegar to lessen the intensity of the heat,and soak for a rotation of 10 minutes on and 10 minutes off.

Sprains (poultice)

Soothe a sprained muscle by wrapping the sore area with a cloth that has been drenched and wrung out of apple cider vinegar. Leave vinegar-laden cloth in place for 5 to 7 minutes, and repeat as needed for relief.

Sprains (poultice again)

The addition of cayenne pepper increases the potency of this poultice. Combine 1/2 cup of apple cider vinegar with 1/4 teaspoon of cayenne pepper in a dish. Soak a soft cloth and wring out any dripping moisture, still keeping the cloth wet. Apply to sore muscle area for 3 to 5 minutes, at least 3 times a day.

Sprains (poultice wrap)

Combine a cup of apple cider vinegar with a tablespoon of baking soda in a small bowl. Soak a clean cloth in the solution and wring out the extra liquid. Apply directly to the sprain in 5 to 10 minute intervals to help reduce swelling and ease pain.

Stomach Digestion Problems

Apple cider vinegar is an effective stabilizer of digestive issues. Combine 1/2 cup of vinegar with 1/4 cup of water and 1 teaspoon of fennel seeds. Warm gently over medium heat to allow the fennel seeds to infuse with the vinegar. Pour into a teacup and enjoy while simultaneously treating the digestive tract. For a sweeter taste, feel free to add a dollop of honey (preferably raw, local honey).

Sunburn

To find relief from the pain of a sunburn, gently splash or spray undiluted apple cider vinegar directly onto burned areas for a cooling effect.

Sunburn Paste

This is another old-time remedy which has been time-tested and approved! Combine 1/8 of a cup of apple cider vinegar with about 1 cup of oatmeal to form a soft paste. More vinegar or oatmeal can be added to make the correct consistency. Gently dab this paste onto sunburned areas of the skin to help ease pain and bring instant relief.

Sunburn Skin Tonic

Combine 1/8 cup of apple cider vinegar with a teaspoon of lemon juice. In a bowl, soak a clean cloth and wring out the extra moisture. Softly apply wet cloth directly to sunburned skin.

Sunburn Soak

One of the most thorough reliefs for all-over sunburn pain is a cooling soak. Pour one half cup of apple cider vinegar into a cool bath. Soak to ease the pain of sunburn and reduce the redness.

Urinary Tract Infection

Vinegar is a natural combatant to urinary tract infections. Its antibacterial and antiseptic properties make it exceptionally effective. Simply consume 1 teaspoon of apple cider vinegar (with or without water) to reduce instances of urinary tract and bladder infections.

Urinary Tract Infection Soak

A secondary approach to dealing with irritating and painful urinary tract infections comes in the form of a soak. Simply add 1 cup of apple cider vinegar to warm bath water and soak for 20 to 30 minutes for infection relief.

Varicose Veins

Try healing varicose veins with this remedy. Combine 1 teaspoon each of apple cider vinegar and honey into a glass of water and consume once or twice a day. You can also consider using this remedy in conjunction with the vinegar poultice remedy that follows for greater effectiveness.

Varicose Veins (poultice)

Here is a two-pronged approach to treating varicose veins.

Soak a clean, soft cloth in undiluted apple cider vinegar. Wring out and place over varicose veins with legs propped up for 30 minutes in both the morning and evening. Considerable relief should be noticed within 6 weeks.

To speed up the healing process, follow each poultice treatment with a glass of warm water to which a teaspoonful of apple cider vinegar has been added. Sip slowly and add a teaspoon of honey, if feeling over tired.

Weight Loss

Weight loss and vinegar have been long associated. In fact, several research studies have been conducted looking into the effectiveness of using vinegar to shed pounds.

Mix 1 teaspoon of apple cider vinegar into a cup of warm water and consume before each meal. This will help moderate an over-active appetite and eliminate fat.

Welts

Blend 1 tablespoon of apple cider vinegar with 1 tablespoon of cornstarch, making a thick paste. Pat paste directly onto itchy, welted area and allow to dry. Gently wash paste from skin using warm water, followed by a cool rinse.

Chapter Three
Beautiful You

W hile the rigorous health benefits of vinegar are well documented throughout recorded history, it is easy to overlook its use as it relates to beauty and skin care. In fact, vinegar's usage as a beauty agent is every bit as cataloged as its more widely known medicinal aspect, going nearly as far back in history as vinegar itself. From the allure and elegance of Cleopatra to the beauty regimen of royalty, vinegar has solidified its place in the annals of cosmetic history.

Vinegar may not actually turn back the hands of time, but scientific research does seem to support claims that it does hold significant benefit to bring cosmetic improvements to the body's skin, nails and hair.

But Does it Really Work?

Scientific studies confirm that apple cider vinegar can be of significant benefit when used to help restore and balance pH levels throughout the body, particularly when it comes to delicate skin and hair issues. Vinegar itself contains a pH level nearly identical to that of healthy human skin, which makes it the obvious choice to correct those type of issue and solve chemical imbalances.

Being a known astringent, apple cider vinegar is an excellent option to many of today's harsher, chemical-based cleansers found on drugstore shelves. It is a logical choice for affording smooth, youthful-looking skin while at the same time restoring the natural elasticity of hair that is so common to lose as we age. Best of all, it can help repair damaged hair and restore luster and shine, all without the use of chemicals which can further deplete hair shafts and follicles of essential nutrients.

Vinegar also contains antioxidant properties which can help fight free radicals. Why is this important? Because research has shown that free radicals cause much of the body's aging and the corresponding damage that reins with it. As free radicals occur as a by-product of the body's own metabolism, they are responsible for a host of diseases and conditions which come with growing older. Some of these, such as arthritis and a weakened immune system, begin a domino effect that is responsible for even more damage. Outwardly, these changes manifest themselves more visibly in the form of wrinkles or spotting of the skin and lifeless hair.

Vinegar is a water-soluble solution that is packed with essential vitamins, minerals and elements crucial to the human body. This makes vinegar stand alone as a natural beauty agent. Some of the most studied and well-documented areas of success using apple cider vinegar include its ability to:

- Balance pH levels in the skin
- Combat pimples and other skin blemishes through its antiseptic properties
- Deodorize naturally
- Soothe dry or damaged skin
- Clean and open skin pores
- Restore youthful skin appearance
- Strengthen and add luster to damaged hair
- Skin detoxification
- Lightening age spots
- Reduce discoloration of nails

For generations, vinegar has been credited with the ability to improve everything from the skin's glowing finish to naturally highlighting hair to bringing calm and comfort to a calming bath. It brings relief and adds beauty gently, with a pleasing aroma. Bottom line, vinegar can make people feel better...and that's what it's all about.

Give a few of these beauty treatments a try, and remember that what works for you may not work for someone else. The key benefit to natural home remedies is that they are personal and unique to each user. So feel free to make modifications, where necessary, to get the best result for your particular circumstance.

Acne

To end troublesome bouts of acne, combine together 1 teaspoon of apple cider vinegar, 1 teaspoon of honey and 1 tablespoon of cornstarch until the ingredients form the consistency of a thick paste. Use this paste on pimples and blackheads by gently rubbing solution into blemishes in a circular motion, and follow with a cool rinse. Pat skin dry. Repeat twice daily.

Age Spots

A sure sign of aging happens when we notice age spots first appearing on our hands and face. Try some this apple cider vinegar-based remedy to lighten them. Combine 2 teaspoons of vinegar with 1 teaspoon of lemon juice. Using a drenched cotton ball, apply the combined liquid directly to spots once or twice a day. Age spots should begin to fade away in a few weeks.

Age Spots (a little more)

The combination of apple cider vinegar and onion can work wonders on unsightly age spots. Just pour a little vinegar into a dish and cut an onion in two. Dab the cut side of the onion into the vinegar and gently rub directly onto age spots once a day. Within a few weeks, you should begin to see age spots disappear.

Armpit Odor

Vinegar is a natural disinfectant and odor eliminator. While its effectiveness as both in cleaning is well known, it is every bit as useful in the elimination of body odor. Best of all, vinegar actually neutralizes odors instead of covering them up with heavy perfumes like many of its storebought counterparts. Saturate a clean cloth or paper towel with a few tablespoons of apple cider vinegar. Use the moistened cloth to clean armpits, but do not rinse. Allow to air dry.

Bath Soak: Herbal

Add chamomile to a vinegar bath, or substitute your favorite herbal vinegar, such as peppermint or ginger vinegar for a refreshing soak. Simply draw a bath of warm water and add 3/4 cup of apple cider vinegar along with 3 tablespoons of chamomile. Swirl around to incorporate and enjoy a relaxing herbal soak for at least 20 minutes, or while the water remains warm.

Bath Soak: Skin Softening

By balancing the skin's pH level, apple cider vinegar restores natural moisture and soft youthfulness to aging skin. Simmer 2 bags of your favorite herbal tea in 1 cup of vinegar on the stovetop for 10 minutes. When warmed, add vinegar tea mixture to an already warm bath water for a soothing, softening skin bath.

Bath Soak: Soothing

In a plastic bottle, combine 1/4 cup apple cider vinegar with 2 tablespoons of your favorite shampoo and 1 cup olive oil. When ready for a soothing soak, add 1/4 cup of this mixture to warm bath water. For a variation, replace apple cider vinegar with tonics such as lavender or woodruff herbal vinegar.

Body Deodorizer

Eliminate body odor with the freshness of vinegar. Combine 1/4 cup apple cider vinegar with 1/4 cup water in a small cup or bowl. Following your shower or bath, use to rub down any high areas of your body and allow to air dry.

Corns and Calluses

The acidity of vinegar can help dissolve painful corns and calluses on contact. Add 1/2 cup of apple cider vinegar to a bucket of warm water and soak feet for 5 minutes. Remove feet from bucket and, while still wet, rub about 1 tablespoon of white table sugar on the bottoms of feet and any area affected by corns or calluses. Massage sugar gently into skin, adding more sugar as necessary. Next, add a bit of baby oil and continue to massage and rub into feet. Finally, wash feet clean with mild soap and water and pat dry. Cover with cotton socks. Repeat daily, as needed.

Dandruff

Try a little vinegar as a hair rinse to put an end to pesky dandruff flakes, and leave the scalp healthy and rejuvenated. Combine 2 teaspoons of apple cider vinegar in a glass bowl filled with 1/4 cup of water. Wet a comb or brush in the vinegar-water solution and brush through hair, especially into the roots. Rub the remaining liquid into the scalp, massage it through as you go along. Allow to set wet on hair for 10 minutes, and then wash as usual.

Dandruff Deep Treatment

Oftentimes a solution to dandruff calls for a more deep treatment. This is a unique treatment meant to not only reduce dandruff flaking, but also stimulate the scalp and growth follicles. In a small bowl, combine together 1/2 cup of apple cider vinegar with 2 pulverized aspirins. Shampoo and rinse hair as usual. Comb the aspirin and vinegar solution through hair and allow to condition hair follicles for 5 minutes, massaging scalp for at least 2 of those minutes of the time. Use fresh water to rinse clean. Next add a second 1/2 cup of vinegar to a quart of warm water and use this as the final rinse for your hair.

Dandruff Rinse

Combine 1/2 cup of apple cider vinegar with 2 cups of warm water in a bowl or dish. After shampooing hair, immediately rinse with vinegar mixture as your final rinse. Style hair as usual. If you prefer to use your own favorite conditioner, you can use this in addition to conditioning as a final, second rinse.

Dandruff Second Rinse

Immediately following your normal routine shampooing and rinsing (or conditioning, if that is what you choose), give hair a second rinse with a solution made of 1/4 cup of apple cider vinegar and 1/4 cup of water.

Dandruff Treatment

For bad bouts of dandruff, daily washing can make the scalp even drier, worsening the condition. As a dandruff treatment effective for daily use, try rubbing a few tablespoons of undiluted apple cider vinegar into the scalp and allow head to air dry. This treatment can be used even if you choose not to wash your hair, and should help to reduce dandruff.

Denture Cleaner

Vinegar possesses numerous qualities that help in the cleaning, disinfecting and deodorizing of dentures. Not only it is highly effective, but can also be used for mere pennies compared to the more expensive commercial choices. You will find several remedies for cleaning dentures. It's up to you to decide which entry works best for you. Either type of vinegar can be used for denture cleaning. White vinegar is a common choice, or apple cider vinegar which leaves a more refreshing twist.

Combine 1/2 teaspoon of your favorite type of vinegar (white or apple cider) with 3/4 cups of water. Drop in dentures and allow to soak overnight.

Denture Cleaner (mint)

For a minty flavor to your denture cleaner, try this remedy. Combine 1 cup of water with 1 teaspoon of white vinegar. Tear several fresh mint leaves into pieces and add to the solution. Place dentures in vinegar water and soak dentures overnight.

Denture Cleaner (whitener)

Dentures have a way of losing their brightness and becoming dull over time. Use your toothbrush to brush a bit of white vinegar directly onto dentures, and gently clean. This will not only remove lingering food odors, but also help restore dentures to their original shine. When finished, rinse and air dry.

Detoxify the Body

Many people swear by vinegar's ability to detoxify the body. The key is in using raw, unfiltered vinegar which still contains the "mother" that is rich is healthful benefits. Simply add 1 or 2 tablespoons of vinegar to a cup of water and drink daily for a short period of time. If the taste is too robust for your liking, a dollop of honey can be added to soften the taste and make it more palatable.

Dry Skin Prevention

Give your skin a boost by preventing dryness before it happens, Mix 1/4 cup apple cider vinegar with 1/4 cup olive oil. Use this combination to apply a protective coating to exposed skin before heading outdoors. This extra moisturizer also prevents chapping during the winter months.

Facial Mask

Use this mask once a week for young, beautiful skin. In a medium bowl, combine 1/2 cup apple cider vinegar with 1/4 cup of oatmeal and 1/4 cup of cooked rice until thoroughly mixed. Pat mixture onto face and neck and allow to dry for about 10 minutes. Gently wash off oatmeal paste with lukewarm water. Next, follow with a second rinse of cool water. Softly pat skin dry with a clean towel.

Deep Facial Mask

Combine 1 tablespoon of apple cider vinegar, 1 tablespoon of honey, 1/2 mashed banana and 1/2 mashed peach in a bowl until it forms a sticky paste. Gently apply to neck and face and allow to set for about 10 minutes. Rinse completely clean and pat dry.

Facial Moisturizing Mask

There are so many combinations of ingredients that work hand in hand with vinegar to make healing facial masks. Combine 1 tablespoon of apple cider vinegar with 1 tablespoon of honey and 1/4 cup of oatmeal. Mix everything together and gently pat onto wet facial skin. Allow to air dry completely, and then rinse away with a cool rinse. Apply your favorite moisturizer.

Facial Steam

Leave your face feeling fresh and looking radiant with a vinegar facial. Heat a cup of vinegar on the stovetop, bringing to a boil. Remove vinegar from stove and carefully pour hot vinegar into a large bowl. Placing a towel over your head, lean over the bowl and cover your head. Allow the warm steam to soften facial skin. Remain with face over bowl until steaming action has ended. After the vinegar has cooled down and you are no longer able to use it for steaming, gently dab a little onto the face and neck as a refreshing cleaning astringent.

Facial Toner

This simple combination works wonders on the skin, without drying. Put a plastic bottle together ahead of time to keep in the bathroom for your morning beauty routine. Just combine 1/2 cup of apple cider vinegar with 1/2 cup of water. Each morning, use a cotton ball to apply to face and neck, and allow to air dry.

Facial Wash

This is a fantastic wash to bring back youthful tenderness to the skin. Mash 3 large strawberries into 1/4 cup of vinegar and leave on the counter undisturbed for 2 hours. Strain strawberry-vinegar solution through a cheesecloth or sieve and discard lumps. Before bed, pat strawberry-flavored vinegar onto face and neck. In the morning, wash solution off face with normal morning cleansing routine.

Fingernail Fungus

To rid nails of fungus, combine 1/2 cup of white vinegar in 1/2 cup of water in a shallow bowl. Soak fingernails for 10 to 15 minutes twice each day and pat dry.

Fingernail Fungus (more)

Saturate a cotton ball with white vinegar and use to wipe down fingernails. Be sure to not only clean the nail itself, but also the nail bed and cuticle area — anywhere fungus could be hiding to grow. Repeat 3 times a day.

Fingernail Polish Prep

Ever wonder why nail polish seems to go on smoother and last longer when it's applied at the salon? Many times the salon preps the nailbed first, making for a prettier end result. You can do this at home with simple vinegar. Try this quick vinegar trick to have your favorite nail polish go on smoother and remain on days longer.

Use a cotton ball to clean uncoated fingernails with about a teaspoon of white vinegar and allow to air dry. Once completely dry, paint nails with your favorite nail polish.

Foot Odor

To eliminate foot odor, soak feet in a pan of about 1 quart of strong, warm tea for 5 to 10 minutes. Combine 1 cup each of apple cider vinegar and warm water. Remove feet from tea soak and rinse with vinegar and water combination. Pat dry as the final step. Repeat as necessary.

Foot Odor

Wipe down feet two times a day with about 1/4 cup of undiluted apple cider vinegar using a cotton balls or a clean cloth. Do not rinse, but allow feet to air dry to remove bothersome odor.

Foot Softener

Add a half cup of apple cider vinegar to a bucket of warm water and soak feet for 10 to 15 minutes. Remove feet and pat dry. Once completely dry, apply your favorite body or foot lotion and cover with a clean pair of socks, allowing your feet to fully absorb the lotion.

Hair Frizz

Dry hair, static and humidity can all wreak havoc on hair, leaving it lifeless and frizzy. To restore hair back to its more healthy, original state, Combine 1/2 cup of apple cider vinegar with 1 cup of warm water in a cup. Shampoo hair as usual, using your favorite conditioner if necessary. For the final rinse, pour warm vinegar water solution through hair and into scalp. Do not rinse away with additional water.

Hair Hot Oil Treatment

This is an excellent treatment to work into your beauty routine on a regular basis. Heat 1/4 cup of olive oil until warm (not hot) and massage into hair. Apply most of the oil through the strands and into the ends of the hair, avoiding the scalp (as the scalp can begin to appear greasy if too much oil remains there). Fill a sink or bowl with hot tap water and add 1/2 cup apple cider vinegar. Soak a bath towel in the vinegar water and then wring it out by hand. Towel should be wet, but not dripping. Wrap the moist, warm towel around hair and allow to soak in for 20 to 30 minutes. Remove towel and wash hair as normal. Repeat once a month, or more often for particularly dry or damaged hair.

Hair Loss

To combat hair loss, keep the follicles rejuvenated and stimulated with this vinegar tonic. Combine 1 teaspoon apple cider vinegar into 3/4 cup of clean water. Drink this mixture every day for 4 to 6 weeks. New hair follicles should begin to appear after that time.

Hair Moisturizer

Give your hair an extra bit of moisturizing treatment with this remedy. Combine 1/4 cup of apple cider vinegar, 2 teaspoonfuls of honey, 1 egg yolk and 1/3 cup olive oil and mix until well incorporated. Gently rub this mixture into your hair and scalp, and then wrap treated hair in a we towel. Allow to set in hair for 10 minutes, and then shampoo out as usual. Next, rinse hair in lukewarm water with an additional 1/4 cup of vinegar added to it for the final rinse.

Hair Richness

As we begin to age, hair naturally loses some of its luster and richness during the aging process. To bring back that youthful look, combine 4 teaspoons of apple cider vinegar, 4 teaspoons of black strap molasses, 4 teaspoons of honey in a cup of water. Begin each day by drinking this concoction to maintain a rich, healthy head of hair.

Hair Rinse

Vinegar makes an excellent final rinse to hair to clean, revitalize and add a natural shine. Combine 1/4 cup of water with 1/2 cup of apple cider vinegar. Following a shower or bath, give hair a final rinse with this vinegar water solution. Leave in hair, without a water rinse, but instead allow to air dry.

Hand Softener

Keep some of this softening solution on hand for days working in the garden or in the garage to restore moisture and softness to overworked hands. Crudely combine 1 teaspoon of vinegar, 1/2 cup of water, 1/2 teaspoon of white sugar with 1 teaspoon of baby oil. Work this mixture into hands for 2 minutes, covering all parts of the hands including backs, palms and between the fingers. Wash clean with a mild soap. Use as part of your daily beauty routine for soft hands, or anytime a little extra softness is needed.

Hand Softener for Overnight Soaking

Add 1 tablespoon apple cider vinegar to 2 cups of warm water and soak hands for 5 minutes. Pat hands dry with a soft cloth or clean towel. Smooth about 1/2 teaspoon of petroleum jelly over hands and cover with a pair of clean cotton gloves. Wear gloves overnight while you sleep, and by morning hands will be unbelievably soft and smooth.

Itchy Skin

Fill a bathtub with warm water and add about 3 cups of apple cider vinegar. Sprinkle a handful of fresh thyme to the water, if desired, and soak in this vinegar bath every day to relieve all-over dry, itchy skin.

Men's Aftershave

This combination contains great natural herbs for men's aftershave. Thyme, sage, bay leaves or cloves can be used to give a rugged, outdoors aroma. Also consider some of the more gently, healing herbs such as bee balm, chamomile and spearmint.

Combine 1 cup of white vinegar with 2 tablespoons of honey and 1 tablespoon of your favorite fresh herb. Mix these together and place in a small jar with a tight fitting lid. Allow to rest undisturbed for up to one week. Open jar and strain out any floating herbs or debris. Now this daily aftershave is ready to use.

Men's Aftershave Cooler

Place 1 small cucumber with its peel in a blender along with a few fresh mint leaves. Puree into a fine consistency. Combine 1 cup of white vinegar with 2 tablespoons of honey and then add the mint puree. Place in a small jar and seal with a lid. Place in refrigerator overnight. In the morning, strain out any cucumber peel or floating herbs with a fine sieve. Pour tonic into a glass or plastic decanter, preferably one using a pump action dispenser, and use daily.

Men's Skin Bracer

Use a touch of distilled vinegar to make your own skin bracer for men. Not only is it clean and refreshing, but vinegar's astringent properties help make it especially healing.

Combine 2 tablespoons of white vinegar with 1/2 teaspoon cream of tartar and 1/3 cup warm water. Wash face as usual and pat dry. Gently pat bracer onto skin.

Mouthwash

Vinegar has been used all across the world as a mouthwash, to kill bacteria and leave the mouth feeling fresh. Both types of vinegars are recommended here, and both do an equally good job with slightly different flavorings. Apple cider vinegar can be used for any healing that needs to take place in the mouth, leaving its familiar robust flavor behind. Distilled vinegar can also be used for a more intense flavor. The choice is yours! And, as with most home remedies, alterations and additions can be made to further personalize the mouthwash into something you will love to use.

Just combine 1 cup of warm water with 2 tablespoons of apple cider or distilled vinegar. Add 1/8 teaspoon of peppermint flavoring (not oil) or any other flavoring you find pleasing. Gargle with solution and rinse mouth clean for a disinfecting, fresh feeling that protects your mouth.

pH Levels in the Skin

One of the best reasons vinegar is used in beauty regimens is its ability to regulate and balance the skin's pH level, leaving your skin silky and soft, and looking younger. This entry is gently enough to use every day, and is as easy as keeping a bottle of apple cider vinegar in your medicine cabinet along with a few soft cotton balls.

Just soak a cotton ball or clean towelette in apple cider vinegar and gently apply to your face and neck to balance alkalines in the skin. In no time, you can see a noticeable difference in the look and feel of your skin. It's also a great addition to your morning beauty routine as a skin toner before applying daily moisturizer or make up.

pH Level Body Wash

There is no reason to just use vinegar to balance pH levels on the face. Your entire body can benefit from a little apple cider vinegar as well. This body was is a great way to leave your skin soft and avoid harsh soaps which can dry out the skin. Just add 1/2 cup of vinegar to 1/2 cup of water and use as rejuvenating splash after bathing. No need to rinse, just allow to air dry or gently pat with a soft towel.

Rectal Itching

Soak a clean gauze pad in 1/8 cup of apple cider vinegar and apply directly onto rectal itch for instant relief. Repeat as necessary.

Skin Lightening

This vinegar and lemon juice combination can not only lighten skin, but does it in such a way that leaves skin feeling fresh and hydrated, not dried out. Combine 1/4 cup of white vinegar, 1/4 cup of lemon juice, 1/2 cup of white wine and 1 tablespoon of honey. Mix until well incorporated, and store in a jar or bottle. Twice each day, gently apply a bit to the face by blotting on with a soft cotton ball or small cloth. Allow to air dry before continuing with normal beauty routine.

Soiled Hands

Wet hands that are heavily soiled with a tablespoon of apple cider vinegar. Sprinkle 1 teaspoon of cornmeal into both hands and rub vigorously together to clean hands and eliminate any lingering odor. Rinse in cool water and pat dry.

Sunburn

Saturate a clean cloth with undiluted apple cider vinegar. Gently place cloth on sunburned area of the skin for instant, cooling relief.

Sunburn Soak

Fill a bathtub with lukewarm water, taking care to not allow temperature to become too hot. Add 1 cup of apple cider vinegar and soak for 15 to 20 minutes for relief of sunburn pain.

Toenail Trimming

Brittle toenails can be difficult to safely trim and file. Try this solution to soften nails immediately prior to trimming. Mix 3 tablespoons of apple cider vinegar with 4 cups of water. Soak feel and toes in solution for 10 minutes, right before cutting nails. Dry feet and proceed to trim and file.

Warts

Soak a pice of cotton gauze or a cotton ball in apple cider vinegar and place directly on top of wart. Tape into place with cloth taping and leave on for 30 minutes. Repeat twice a day until the wart is gone.

Weight Loss

Research studies have shown that apple cider vinegar may, in fact, aid in weight loss by several way. It may not only boost metabolism and suppress the appetite, but also burn calories through thermogenics. Try this simple solution to start shedding pounds immediately. Stir 2 teaspoons of apple cider vinegar into a glass of water. Drink 20 minutes before mealtime to shed extra pounds.

Wrinkles

Combine 1/4 cup apple cider vinegar with 1 tablespoon of fennel seeds and heat over medium heat until hot. Turn the heat down and allow to simmer uncovered for 30 minutes, allowing some of the moisture to evaporate out. Remove from heat and cool completely. Pour into a jar with a tight-fitting lid.

Saturate a cotton ball with fennel-infused vinegar and gently dab over face and neck. For even greater soothing action, gently heat jar of fennel vinegar in microwave before using. Test to be sure vinegar is warm and not hot. Use warm vinegar and fennel combination to dab over wrinkles. This warmed version allows for greater moisturizing penetration. Use once or twice a day.

Chapter Four
Cleaning with Vinegar

Vinegar's reputation as a potent cleaning agent and disinfect has been recognized for generations. Not only does it carry a reputation for being one of the best, most versatile cleaning solutions available, it works for just pennies on the dollar, leaves no toxic residues behind and is friendly to the environment. And best of all, there appears to be ample scientific research to back up these claims.

But first, what makes vinegar so potent as a household cleaner, and how can we best harness its effectiveness?

What Makes Vinegar Special?

Vinegar has already been well established as a home remedy aid to literally hundreds of conditions and ailments. Many of these same properties contribute to elevate vinegar as a workhorse of a cleaning agent. Vinegar is both antibacterial and antiseptic in nature, which allows it to not only eliminate harmful bacteria on contact, but also inhibit bacteria's ability to return. Simply put, once an area has been disinfected with vinegar, germs have a difficult time regrouping on the same area. This makes surfaces vinegar comes in contact with not only clean to the naked eye, but the underlying bacteria has also been removed.

Ironically, vinegar's ability to pull calcium from chicken bones in cooking recipes, for example, is the same trait which allows it to successfully dissolve harsher stains and breakup built up deposits... but safely. Since vinegar is gently enough to consume, it lacks the toxic effects you may find with store bought cleaning supplies.

Because vinegar is an acid-based solution, it is exceptionally powerful when it comes to removing difficult types of stains, such as mineral deposits or microscopic particles, that many commercial cleaners can't touch. It is considered an all-purpose cleaner which is successful in not only cleaning difficult rust stains, but also delicate enough for china and crystal. In short, it is the perfect go-to product for a wide gamut of cleaning endeavors.

Vinegar's composition is a very strong, non-toxic liquid that is ideal for breaking down deposits such as calcium carbonate and other mineral-based deposits. These microscopic particles which are commonly found in hard water areas of the country can adhere to household plumbing and drains and eventually build up causing plumbing and drainage problems. The acidity in vinegar is potent, get gentle enough, to remove these deposits without harming pipes, unlike many chemical cleaners.

Vinegar is Safer to Use, and Gentle on the Environment

Commercial cleaning solvents contain a host of chemicals which can be harmful to both the human body and to the environment. And when these same cleaning agents are combined with other chemical-based products, the result can be toxic. Many of store bought products release harmful fumes, but also leave toxic residue behind on the very items they "cleaned. Studies have also been conducted to research whether the chemicals themselves may be more dangerous than the bacteria they were manufactured to eliminate.

There is also the very real complication regarding the disposal of these chemicals after use. Most are poured down drains, discarded in sanitation bins or flushed down the toilets. The problem occurs when these compounds reach and contaminate the environment in the form of delicate streams and waterways, in addition to filling landfills with not only the toxins themselves, but the bottles and jars they are stored in. A less discussed issue is in the manufacture of these products, which in itself is harsh on the environment through chemicals released during production.

Vinegar, on the other hand, is completely natural. It is not only the chemical-free choice for potent cleaning, but also safe for the environment and biodegradable, helping to keep our natural resources like riverbeds and streams clean. It can be purchased for pennies on the dollar, which makes it a solid economical choice compared to store bought cleaners.

Being all-natural, vinegar is also safe for use around small children and pets. It is even used to clean up after infants. After all, vinegar can be eaten. How many commercial cleaners can boast that fact?

What Type of Vinegar Works Best for Cleaning?

For most cleaning applications, both distilled and apple cider vinegar can do the job well. Due to the greater volume used in cleaning, white vinegar is much less expensive for cleaning purposes, allowing you to use it liberally without financial considerations.

For specific cleaning of light-colored fabrics, it is usually best to stick with distilled vinegar to avoid any chance of staining delicate fabrics. Other times, you may choose apple cider vinegar due to its aromatic fragrance. The choice is yours.

Vinegar's Special Cleaning Considerations

Like all good things, vinegar does have its limitations, and a few cautions go hand in hand with those limitations. While vinegar is a strong choice for cleaning virtually anything, there are a few instances where the use of vinegar should be avoided:

- pearls
- silver
- blood stains
- vomit
- butter
- eggs
- milk

- grease (vinegar is an excellent option for cutting grease, but not for removing grease stains)

Just like any cleaning solution you are using for the very first time, it would be wise to test an inconspicuous area for sensitivity before use. Also, when using vinegar for cleaning substances such as tarnished copper, take great care in the proper disposal of the cleaning rags, as the buffed out green tarnish is poisonous.

Getting the Most out of Cleaning with Vinegar

The following pages contain some of the most effective cleaning solutions around, used on nearly every surface imaginable. To get the most out of these listings, you may wish to mix some of your favorites well ahead of time and save them for future use. Plastic bottles with spray nozzles can be very helpful to put together in advance, along with a selection of common household items to keep nearby to make cleaning easier. Placing these in a small bucket would keep all the items within easy reach, along with a bucket to get the jobs started.

Some of these items might include:

- plastic spray bottles filled and labeled with various vinegar cleaning solutions
- Small fine mist sprayer
- Discarded toothbrush for cleaning small, hard-to-reach areas
- Cotton swabs
- Soft cleaning rags, towels and/or sponges
- Nylon scrubbers
- Scrub brushes
- Paper towels

One simple way to prepare vinegar for cleaning use is to purchase plastic spray caps, or buy a plastic spray bottle and remove its sprayer, and place directly onto a purchased bottle of vinegar. It's simple and ready to use with ease. Remember that the plastic bottles of vinegar are significantly lighter than its glass counterpart, and would work better for this use. In addition, plastic bottles are shatterproof when dropped by slippery hands.

Enjoy experimenting with different vinegar mixtures and techniques. Grab your bucket and supplies, it's time to get started...

Bathrooms

Ceramic Tile

Ceramic tile and bathroom grout can benefit greatly from the powerful cleaning of vinegar. Not only does vinegar clean and disinfect grimy bathroom tile with its disinfection properties, but can also remove soap scum and hard water mineral deposits. In addition, vinegar can help bring stained grout back to its original beauty.

Combine 1/4 cup white vinegar with 1 cup of water. Using a cloth or sponge, wipe down ceramic tile. Follow with a little undiluted white vinegar to clean grout with a toothbrush. When finished, dry thoroughly with a clean towel.

Chrome and Brass Fixtures

In a sink or small bucket, combine 1/2 cup white vinegar with 2 cups of warm water. Using a soft cloth, clean chrome and brass with vinegar-water solution. Dry completely with a clean, soft cloth. Apply 2 applications of a light wax to coat and shine metal. Coating will not only make fixtures shine, but also prevent future build up of hard water deposits and make future cleaning even easier.

Exhaust Fans

Exhaust fans can benefit doubly from a good vinegar cleaning. Not only will vinegar clean and disinfect, but will also rid the fans of any built up odor leaving it fresh for the next use.

First, wipe and clean exhaust fan grill cover being certain to remove any dust and debris. Then, using a clean cloth wet with white vinegar, wipe down the grill cover coating it well to keep dust from reaccumulating on fan grill.

Mirrors

Using a bottle and sprayer, spray white vinegar directly onto a clean cloth. Use cloth to wipe mirror into a streak-free shine. Never spray vinegar, or any other liquid solution, directly onto mirrors. Stray moisture can make its way into the silver backing and destroy the mirror by leaving black marring.

Odors

Bathrooms, left unchecked, can rapidly become a haven for unwanted odors. Vinegar is the perfect solution, not only eliminating odors and keeping the room fresh, but actually neutralizing the source.

Fill a small spray bottle with 1 tablespoon of white vinegar and about 1/2 cup of water. Use a few sprays of this natural deodorizer in the place of aerosol air fresheners to effectively eliminate lingering bathroom odors. This is a great solution to spray at the end of your scheduled bathroom cleaning regimen, or to place in a more decorative spray bottle and keep on hand to freshen the room after each use, as necessary of course!

Shower Curtains

Remove shower curtain from hooks and place in bathtub or wash tub. Fill tub with just enough warm water to completely cover shower curtain. Pour in 2 cups of white vinegar and allow curtain to soak in vinegar water for at least 4 hours, or overnight if possible. In the morning, add 2 tablespoons of liquid dish detergent to vinegar water and wash curtain in tub. Rinse curtain and hang outside to dry in the afternoon sun.

Glass Shower Doors

Combine 1/4 cup white vinegar and 1 teaspoon of alum together. Liberally wipe this mixture on glass shower door and scrub in a circular motion with a soft cleaning brush. Rinse with hot water. Buff with a soft cloth until completely dry.

Shower Door and Mildew

Use this method to remove mildew and scum that build up over time on bathroom shower doors. Dip an old toothbrush into undiluted white vinegar and use scrub out corners and hard-to-reach crevices of the shower door. Next, fill a spray bottle with white vinegar and use to thoroughly wet entire shower door. Wipe clean with a cloth again saturated in vinegar. Rinse clean and towel dry.

Shower Head

Shower heads, with all of their openings and pinpoint nozzles, can be difficult to clean properly. Vinegar allows for some unique cleaning options without worry of chemical interactions, or leaving store bought chemicals on items that may corrode to involve heavy unwanted fumes. Following are several suggestions for cleaning and disinfecting tough mineral deposits from shower heads.

Soak paper towels in white vinegar until fully saturated. Wrap saturated paper towels tightly against the shower head. Do not wring out paper towels. Place plastic bag around coated shower head and secure in place with a rubber band. Leave to soak overnight.

In the morning, remove plastic bag and paper towels and discard. Use a scrub brush with additional vinegar and brush away any remaining scales.

Shower Head Scrubbing

Combine 1/2 cup of white vinegar with 2/3 cup of water. Use a soft cleaning brush to scrub away any mineral build up on bathroom shower heads. This is a great method to incorporate into your weekly bathroom cleaning routine to keep shower heads running clean.

Shower Head Deep Clean

Unscrew the shower head and place in a sink with enough undiluted white vinegar to cover shower head. Allow to soak for 30-45 minutes, more if necessary. Remove shower head and gently brush with a cleaning brush. Use a toothpick or nail to clean out small openings, if blocked. Scrub around openings with an old toothbrush. Rinse in hot water. Dry to a shine with a buffing towel and replace.

Toilet Stains

Pour 1 cup of white vinegar over stained porcelain toilet. Sprinkle 1 cup of borax over wet vinegar stain and let soak undisturbed for 2 hours. Brush with a toilet brush and flush away.

Soap Scum Removal

Combine 1/2 cup of white vinegar, 1/2 cup of ammonia and 3 tablespoons of baking soda together, and stir into a thick paste. Spread paste over soap scum and allow to set for at least 10 minutes. Gently scrub with a cleaning brush. Rinse with a bucket of cool water to which and additional 1/4 cup of vinegar has been added. After removing soap scum from shower and door, use a soap film preventative (next entry) to keep from returning.

Soap Film Preventative

Use this solution as a preventative method to keep soap film and scum from forming on bathroom showers and tubs. Fill a plastic spray bottle with 1 cup of white vinegar and about 1 quart of water. Once a week, spray down shower and tub area to prevent soap film from building up in tub area.

Soap Film Removal

In a bowl, combine 1/2 cup of white vinegar and 1 cup of baking soda into a creamy paste, adding additional vinegar if needed. Spread paste over soap film in shower and allow to set for 10 minutes. Use a soft brush to clean film. Rinse with warm bucket of water to which 1/4 cup of vinegar has been added. Use a soft cloth to buff dry.

Kitchens

Appliances

Combine 1/4 cup of white vinegar, 1 teaspoon of borax and 2 cups of hot water into a spray bottle. Spray vinegar solution on greasy smears on kitchen appliances. Buff in a circular motion with a soft cloth until clean and shiny.

Black Appliances

Just like stainless steel appliances, black or dark colored appliances seem to show every fingerprint or sponge, and can be especially difficult to clean without marring. They show every fingerprint and smudge. They also tend to show swirl markings from cleaning. Try this formula to keep black appliances looking new and smudge free.

Clean your dark appliance as usual. Then, using undiluted white vinegar on a soft, lint-free cloth, do a final wipe down of the appliance. Finish buffing with a dry, soft clean cloth.

Can Openers

Begin by making certain electric can openers are unplugged. Wipe down appliance with a soft cloth dipped in white vinegar. Removable opener blades can also be soaked in a small bowl of undiluted vinegar to loosen and remove any encrusted food, then carefully wipe clean. Next, use a vinegar-soaked cotton swab tip to clean the can opener vents and operation buttons. Finally, wipe dry with a clean cloth.

Coffee Pots

Fill a coffee pot with water and add 1 tablespoon of white vinegar. Allow to set for 10 minutes, and then rinse well.

Coffee Pot Run Through Clean

Combine 1 cup of white vinegar with 1 cup of fresh water. Run this combination through an automatic coffee pot's brewing cycle to clean and freshen.

More Coffee Pot Cleaning

In coffee pot receptacle, pour 1 tablespoon of white vinegar and 2 or 3 drops of detergent. Run one pot of water through a full brewing cycle. Rinse pot several times with hot water.

Automatic Dishwashers

When cleaning automatic dishwashers, be careful to not completely dry the inside bottom of the appliance. Some manufacturers depend on a small amount of moisture remaining in the bottom to keep seals from drying out and cracking.

Pour 2 cups of undiluted white vinegar into the bottom of an empty dishwasher. Run appliance without using any of your regular detergent, only the vinegar. When both wash and rinse cycles end, but before drying cycle begins, turn off dishwasher and with a cleaning cloth wipe down the interior top of the appliance, along with sides and door.

Electric Knives

Make sure the electric knife is not plugged in. Wipe knife with a cloth dampened with undiluted white vinegar and a little soapy water. Saturate area around the dirty blade mounting and allow to set for 5 minutes to loosen grime. Use a toothpick to scrape area clean. Then, wipe electric cord and dry thoroughly before using.

Exhaust Fan Grill

Wash exhaust fan grill, removing any dust and debris. Wet a clean cloth with white vinegar and wipe down the fan grill to remove any remaining grease. This will also work to help retard any future grease build up.

Garbage Disposal

To keep garbage disposals running efficiently and odor free, run a tray of ice cubes down the disposal along with 1/2 cup of white vinegar poured over them each week.

Garbage Disposal Cubes

Freeze a tray of white vinegar "ice" cubes. Keep them on hand to run down the garbage disposal periodically to easily eliminate odors and keep disposal blades sharp.

Garbage Disposal and Drain Deodorizer

Pour 1/4 cup of baking soda down kitchen drain and follow with about 1/2 cup of white vinegar. Allow to set in drain for at least ten minutes. Next, throw in a few ice cubes and run disposal while cold water is running to thoroughly clean and deodorize.

Microwave Ovens

Pour 3 tablespoons of aromatic apple cider vinegar and 1 cup of water into a microwave-safe cup or bowl and place in the microwave. Bring vinegar-water mixture to a boil, and allow to set in a closed microwave for 5 to 10 minutes. Microwave will smell fresh and vinegar-clean.

Microwave Oven Dried Food Removal

In a small, microwave-safe bowl, heat 1/2 cup of white vinegar with 1/2 cup of water in the microwave until it begins to boil. Next, run the microwave on its highest setting for 30 seconds. Using a soft, dampened cloth, spills and baked-on goods should wipe down with ease.

For any additional cleaning, use a soft cloth and the rest of the vinegar solution (once it cools) to wipe away grime.

Mixers

Saturate a clean cloth with white vinegar and wrap cloth around the mixer. Allow to set for 5 minutes. Remove vinegar-soaked cloth and wipe clean.

Ovens

Ovens can get plagued with baked on food items that build up over time. Not only can this change the taste and smells of foods being baked, but can also become a fire hazard if left unchecked. This cleaning method will restore your oven to a surface-clean state.

When using ammonia, you may wish to use rubber or plastic cleaning gloves to protect your hands.

Pour 3 cups of water into a shallow baking dish and place in the oven. Heat to 300ºF. Turn off oven and allow water to remain in a warm oven for 30 minutes, steaming the oven. After 30 minutes, remove baking dish and discard water. Replace with 2 cups of ammonia and place back into warm oven (keeping oven turned off) and allow to set overnight.

In the morning, pour out all ingredients except for 1/2 cup of ammonia. Add 1/2 cup of white vinegar and 2 cups of baking soda to remaining ammonia. Use this mixture to wash down oven surfaces and then allow to set on oven surfaces for 30 minutes. After 30 minutes, wipe away oven cleaner and rinse with clean water. Dry with a towel.

Oven Racks

Remove racks from the oven and spray thoroughly with white vinegar (you may wish to spray the racks outdoors to keep mess in the kitchen to a minimum). Allow racks to air dry. Place racks in a tub of very hot water, 1 cup of vinegar and 1 tablespoon of dish detergent. Let racks soak for 30 minutes. Turn racks and repeat on opposite end if you are unable to fit the entire rack in the tub at one time, so that the entire rack has soaked for a minimum of 30 minutes. You may need to soak racks a second time for more difficult, hard-to-remove debris. Wipe down racks with a cloth or sponge for final cleaning.

Refrigerators

Use this trick to remove any dirt or grease layer that has built up on the top of your refrigerator, one of the most overlooked areas of kitchen.

Spray undiluted white vinegar on top of the refrigerator and add a few drops of your favorite liquid detergent. Using a cloth or sponge, give the entire appliance top a quick pat to make sure vinegar and detergent is in contact with any grease build up. Allow to soak for 15 minutes. Wipe clean with cloth or sponge. Rinse with hot water and a tablespoon or two of additional vinegar and dry completely.

Refrigerators and Freezer Gaskets

Squirt a little liquid detergent into 2 cups of water and use to wipe down refrigerator and freezer gaskets. Next, use some white vinegar to wipe away any mold that may have accumulated. Rinse with clean water and dry with a clean towel.

Refrigerators, Self-Defrosting

Remove the water collection tray and wash in hot, soapy water. Dry tray and replace. Add about 1 tablespoon of white vinegar of the collection tray to retard any growth of bacteria and keep refrigerator smelling fresh and clean.

Small Appliances

When cleaning any small appliance, be certain not to spray any type of liquid solution directly onto the appliance. Keep moisture from entering the appliance's vent to protect internal parts from damage. Appliances should always be unplugged prior to cleaning.

Wipe down appliance with a clean cloth saturated with white vinegar. Use a second clean cloth to buff appliance dry.

Small Appliance Buttons

Saturate the tip of a cotton swab with a little white vinegar, and use to clean tops and around the sides of hard-to-clean appliance buttons and control knobs.

Small Appliance Cords

Wet a soft cloth with white vinegar and use to periodically wipe down appliance cords to keep free from food and other debris that may have collected. Dry with a separate dry cloth.

Stove Tops

Combine 1/2 cup of white vinegar with 1/2 cup of water and 1 teaspoon of liquid detergent. Using a soft cloth, wipe down stove tops to rid cooked on food and grease. Rinse clean with a cloth wet with water and then buff dry.

Stove Tops with Gas Grates

On a stove top, place a pot of water containing 1 or 2 cups of white vinegar. Place individual iron grates from a gas stove in vinegar water. Bring to a boil for 10 minutes. Remove and wipe clean and dry.

Countertops

Wipe down all kitchen countertops and work surfaces with white vinegar on a paper towel to clean, disinfect and prevent mold.

Countertop Cleaner

Combine 1 cup white vinegar with 1 cup water and store in a plastic spray bottle. Use this solution to wipe down kitchen countertops as needed. Make a bottleful of this natural cleaner ahead of time to keep on hand each time you clean the kitchen.

Countertop Scrubber

Keep this scrubber on had for easy cleaning that will not damage countertop surfaces. Completely soak some nylon hosiery in white vinegar. Use this vinegar-laden scrubber to clean difficult areas of kitchen countertops.

Countertop Stains

Soak a paper towel in white vinegar. Lay the soaked paper towel on the caked area and allow to set for 30 to 60 minutes, then wipe clean.

Countertop Disinfectant

Countertops can be a natural magnet for germs and bacteria. Try this to keep kitchen counters free from germs.

Combine 3 tablespoons of white vinegar, 1 teaspoon of liquid soap, 1/2 teaspoon of oil and 1/2 cup of water. Using a wash towel, wipe down kitchen countertops thoroughly to disinfect. This is a particularly effective wipe after handling meats and poultry.

Countertop Stain Remover

Combine 1/4 cup white vinegar with 1/4 cup water and use to wipe down stained counter. For more difficult stains, consider sprinkling a little baking soda on top of counter and wipe clean with this same vinegar combination.

Cutting Boards and Cutting Blocks

Cutting boards and blocks can trap harmful bacteria after use. Wipe down boards with undiluted apple cider vinegar to clean, disinfect and absorb any lingering food odors.

Cutting Boards and Cutting Blocks Deeper Disinfecting

It is imperative to always keep wooden cutting boards and blocks clean and disinfected from the foods they come in contact with. Sprinkle 1 tablespoon of baking soda over wooden cutting board or block and gently rub into the wood. Now spray the baking soda-covered board with white vinegar and allow to stand for 5 minutes. Rinse with clean water, allowing solution to bubble. Rinse an wipe away any remaining solution. Dry wood thoroughly to prevent warping.

Cutting Boards Deep Sanitation

Apply 2 or 3 tablespoons of salt to coat a cutting board, using more if necessary. Allow to rest for 10 minutes. Scrub salt with about 1/2 cup of white vinegar and rinse well using hot water. Dry completely with a soft cloth. For wood cutting boards, it is helpful to occasionally rub in a little vegetable oil to prevent cracking and keep the wood looking like new.

Deodorizer

Soak a clean cloth in apple cider vinegar and wring out any excess moisture. Place the wet cloth on top of a heat or air register and allow air to circulate through moistened cloth for at least 30 minutes to make kitchen smell fresh and odor free.

Deodorizer Pump

Fill a pump bottle with vinegar. Immediately after cooking heavily aromatic dishes, such as fish, cabbage or for boil overs, spray a few pumps of white vinegar in the air to neutralize the odor.

Deodorizer for Cooking Odors

Simmer 1/4 cup of your choice of apple cider vinegar or white vinegar in an uncovered pot of water to clear the air of lingering cooking odors. You will get two very different aromas, depending upon your choice.

For a clean smell, white vinegar may work best. For a special air-freshened scent, try using apple cider vinegar with 1 teaspoon of cinnamon added.

Drains

To keep drains smelling fresh and clean, be sure to use vinegar to neutralize building odors. It is as simple as pouring 1/2 cup of white vinegar down each drain weekly to not only keep drains fresh, but to discourage clogging. No need to rinse away.

Drain Freshener

Pour 1/2 cup of baking soda down the drain, followed by 1/2 cup of undiluted white vinegar. Allow to rest in drain for 10 minutes, then run hot water down drain to rinse clean again.

Drains and Septics

Use this solution once a month to keep drains running free and give a good bacteria boost to septic systems. It also will help cleanse away any lingering odors.

Using 1 package of dry yeast and 2/3 cup of brown sugar, treat each drain in the house. After treating drains, proceed to also treat the septic tank by pouring yeast and brown sugar into a toilet and flushing the tank twice.

Doing this monthly will help keep the drain and septic system running efficiently for many years.

Faucets and Fixtures

Mix 1 tablespoon of white vinegar and 1 tablespoon of cream of tartar into a paste. Rub this paste onto dingy faucets and kitchen fixtures and allow them to dry completely. Then, using a pan of warm water, wash dried paste off of all fixtures and buff dry again with a clean cloth.

Faucets and Fixtures Shine

Combine 1/3 cup of white vinegar with 2/3 cup of water. Using a soft, clean cloth, polish and shine faucets and fixtures.

Garbage Disposal

Freshen a garbage disposal with this weekly treatment. Dump a tray of ice cubes down the kitchen drain and pour 1/2 cup of white vinegar overtop. Run fresh water over ice and vinegar while simultaneously running disposal to clean and freshen.

Garbage Disposal Cubes

This is an excellent trick to keep your disposal in tip top shape!

Combine vinegar and water and fill ice cube tray. Freeze cubes. Frozen vinegar cubes can be stored in a plastic zip bag in the freezer for easy future use.

Just grind a handful of these vinegar cubes in the garbage disposal each week to keep blades sharp and the disposal system odor free.

Dishes, Knives, Etc.

Aluminum Pots and Pans

Pour 1/2 cup white vinegar and about 2 cups clean water into a dirty aluminum pan. Bring this liquid combination to boil over medium heat on the stove top. Remove pan from heat and allow to rest for a few minutes. Carefully pour out the entire solution and now easily wipe the pan clean.

Aluminum Pots and Pans Stains

For tougher stains, combine 1 tablespoon of white vinegar with 1 teaspoon baking soda and mix until it forms a soft paste. Using a paper towel or soft cloth, use this paste to clean and remove stains from aluminum pans by applying directly to stain. Using a circular motion, rub stains lightly from the cookware.

Aluminum Pots and Pans Heavy Stains

Try this tougher solution for heavy and hard to clean stains on your cookware. Combine 1 tablespoon of white vinegar with 1 teaspoon each of baking soda and cream of tartar. Mix these into a thick paste. Rubbing in a circular motion, remove stains from pots and pans. Rinse away any remaining paste once finished.

Aluminum Pots and Pans More Heavy Stains

Here is another solution for heavily stained pots and pans that do not seem to come clean with normal washing. Combine 1 tablespoon of white vinegar with 1 teaspoon each of your favorite liquid dish detergent, baking soda and cream of tartar. This should form a gritty gel once combined. Spread gel over the stains in the pan and rub in a circular motion using a nylon scrubbing pad. The gel can also be left in place for a few minutes between rubbing action. Repeat this a second time, if necessary, and be sure to rinse clean with fresh water.

Ceramic Baking Dishes

Pour about 1/8 cup of white vinegar into a small bowl. Using a nylon scrubber, gently remove baked-on food from ceramic bakeware. Hand or dishwasher wash, as usual.

Copper and Brass Cleaner

Combine 1/4 cup white vinegar with 1/4 cup lemon juice in a small bowl. Using a soft cloth or paper towel, apply this mixture directly onto copper or brass, and clean using a circular motion. Using a clean, soft cloth, buff to a beautiful shine.

One important note about cleaning copper and brass: always be sure to properly discard cleaning rags and paper towels after cleaning. Brass and copper can give way to harmful chemical residue that needs to be disposed of.

Copper Pan Cleaner

With the onset of popular cable cooking shows, copper pans have become more and more popular. They are a fantastic way to cook, but can also sometimes be difficult to clean. Keep your investment looking like new and free from stains with this method.

In a medium sized bowl, mix 1 cup white vinegar, 1/2 cup powdered dish detergent, 1/2 cup water, 1/2 cup salt and 1/4 cup flour, whisking thoroughly until well blended. Heat slowly in a double boiler until detergent is dissolved and mixture begins to thicken. Remove from heat and cool completely. Once cool, use this mixture to wipe onto a copper pot and coat. Allow coating to rest for 1 to 3 minutes, and wipe clean with a soft cloth. Dampen cloth, if necessary. Once clean, buff with a second cloth to a high shine.

Enamel Baking Dishes

Wash all easy-to-remove food from enamel baking dish. Pour 2 cups of white vinegar, or enough to cover baked on food, into the dish. If 2 cups is not enough, add more as needed. Place baking dish on stovetop or in oven and bring vinegar to a boil in the dish. Continue to boil for several minutes before removing from heat and allow to cool completely. Pour out vinegar and wash baking dish as usual. Baked-on foods should now easily come off.

When pouring out the discarded vinegar, it is a good opportunity to rinse away and freshen odor-filled kitchen sinks and drains.

Fine China

Fine china should always be washed by hand, and never in the dishwasher, to avoid chips and breaks. Note: This solution is for china that is free from gold or silver trim. Vinegar is known to cause metal trim work to discolor, and should be avoided.

Gently wash the fine china by hand in warm, soapy water. Rinse clean in a sink full of hot water to which about 1/4 cup of white vinegar has been added. Dry each piece of china with a clean, soft cloth. To store safely, place a paper plate or paper towel between each delicate piece to prevent any chance of chipping or cracking.

Glassware

Add 1/4 cup of white vinegar to the final rinse water for dishes. After washing glassware, soak each piece in hot vinegar water for a few minutes. Remove, and allow to air dry for clean, streak-free glasses.

Grease Cutter

Add 1/2 cup white vinegar to dishwater along with your favorite dish soap as usual. The added vinegar will work to cut heavy grease in the water for cleaner dishes.

Lead Crystal

Lead crystal, just like fine china, should always be washed by hand, and never in an automatic dishwasher.

Make a sink full of warm, soapy water using your favorite liquid detergent. Place a rubber tub mat in the bottom of the sink to keep lead crystal safe from chips and scratches. Submerge each piece of lead crystal into the soapy water and wash thoroughly. Rinse in a sink full of hot water to which 1/4 cup of white vinegar has been added. Place crystal on a clean towel or drying rack and allow to air dry.

Musty Glass Jars

Dampen a clean sponge with undiluted white vinegar and wring out most of the excess. Place the dampened sponge in the glass jar and seal tightly with the lid. Leave undisturbed allowing the treated sponge to soak up musty odors for at least an hour before removing. Wash jar as usual.

Non-Stick Pans

This solution will help remove mineral deposits and other difficult stains from non-stick coated cookware without damaging its coating.

Pour 2 cups water and 1/3 cup white vinegar into a non-stick pan stained with mineral deposits. Bring to a boil over medium heat on a stovetop. Allow to boil for 3 to 5 minutes. Carefully discard solution and wipe pan clean with a soft cloth.

Pewter

This is an old-time cleaning tip that dates back generations. Soak cabbage leaves in about 3 tablespoons of white vinegar. Dip wet cabbage leaf in a teaspoon of salt and use to clean and buff pewter. Rinse with cool, clean water and dry with a soft cloth.

Pewter Cleaner

Combine 1 tablespoon white vinegar with 1 tablespoon each of salt and flour, adding just enough water to form a soft paste. Smear paste onto discolored pewter and allow to dry completely. Rub off dried paste with a soft cloth or paper towel. Rinse in hot water and buff completely dry.

Greasy Pots and Pans

Place undiluted white vinegar in a spray bottle. Spray a thick coating of vinegar on greasy pots and pans. Allow to set 3-5 minutes. Grease should now wash off much easier, using less dish soap and elbow grease!

Greasy, Stuck-on Food

Combine 1/2 cup white vinegar with 1 and 1/2 cups of warm water. Pour into dirty pot with stuck-on food. Heat vinegar and water mixture in dirty pot until very warm. Discard the water and wipe pan clean.

Thermoses

Use this trick to clean thermoses that are hard to clean due to narrow openings. Combine 1 cup white vinegar and 1/2 cup water and use it to fill thermos. Fit with lid and shake to coat entire inside of thermos. Let stand for 1 hour. After an hour, add about 1 tablespoon of uncooked rice and shake for an additional 2 minutes. Pour out contents and rinse thoroughly. Air dry.

Vases with Narrow Openings

Odd-shaped flower vases can be difficult to clean due to their shape and narrow openings. Try this trick to help clean even the most difficult-shaped vase.

Pour 1/4 cup of uncooked rice into the vase opening, using a funnel if needed. Follow rice with 1/2 cup white vinegar and 1/2 cup of cold water. Shake vase, spinning it in a circular motion, then in reverse direction to loosen grime or dirt. Let set for 1 minute and repeat shaking and swirling action. Pour out rice and vinegar solution. Rinse out vase with 1/4 cup of white vinegar and 1/3 cup warm water. Empty contents and set upside down on countertop and allow to air dry.

Vases

Pour 1/8 cup white vinegar into a small dish. Use a nylon scrub brush dipped in vinegar to clean hard-to-reach areas of the vase's interior. Rinse with hot water and air dry.

More Vases

Pour 3 tablespoons of sand into vase opening. Follow with 1/4 cup each of white vinegar and hot water. Shake or swirl vase vigorously, removing dirt deposits from inside of vase. Empty all contents from vase and rinse well before drying.

Vase Waterlines

Soak a paper towel with undiluted white vinegar and use this to wipe down inside of vase to remove lingering waterlines.

Sharp Knives

Spray undiluted white vinegar onto the bottom of a clay pot until wet. Sharpen dull kitchen knives by using clay pot as a whetstone.

Sponges

Rinse dirty kitchen sponges in the sink and wring out excess. Place 4 cups of water and 1/4 cup white vinegar in a bucket and add sponges to solution. Allow to soak clean overnight to remove dirt and lingering odors before wringing out. No need to rinse; allow to air dry.

Flooring

Carpet Cleaning

As with any new cleaning method, particularly on fabrics, be sure to test a small area of the carpet for colorfastness prior to cleaning larger areas.

Combine 1 cup of white vinegar and 1 gallon of water together and pour into a spray bottle. Spray carpet in areas that are in most need of cleaning, saturating carpet and allowing to soak in for several minutes. Wipe clean with an absorbent cloth or towel. If stain is persistent, repeat a second time, doing so before carpet has had an opportunity to dry.

Carpet Stains

Combine 1/2 cup white vinegar and 2 tablespoons of salt until a soft paste forms. Rub paste into carpet stain and allow to dry completely. It is very important to make sure paste is completely dry and not damp (you may run the risk of clogging or damaging your vacuum cleaner). Vacuum up stain and chalky residue with vacuum and finish vacuuming floor.

Carpet Stains, Heavy

Dissolve 2 tablespoons of salt and 2 tablespoons of borax into 1/2 cup of white vinegar. Rub solution into heavily soiled carpet stain and allow to air dry completely. After solution is dry, use vacuum cleaner to easily sweep up any stain and chalky residue that is left behind.

Carpet Stained by Water

This is an excellent solution to remove stains from carpet that has become wet or flooded, and has left a stain from its own carpet backing.

Combine 1/4 cup white vinegar with 1 cup of water. Wet the stain with the vinegar and water solution, and blot dry with a paper towel or clean rag. Repeat, if necessary, until water stain is gone.

This is especially helpful for water stains created from gentle flooding or broken pipes. The vinegar not only helps remove the stain, but disinfects the area from bacteria that may be left behind.

Floor Cleaner

Combine 1/2 cup white vinegar, 1/4 cup liquid soap, 1/4 cup lemon juice and 2 gallons of water in a large, clean bucket. Use this combination to wash and brighten floors during your weekly cleaning routine.

Floor Cleaner for Wax Build Up

Vinegar is a great solution for dissolving preexisting wax on floors that has built up. Use small amounts to achieve clean and shine. Move to a higher concentration to remove heavy, built up wax where dirt has become ingrain and dulled the flooring.

Add 1 cup white vinegar to a bucket of soapy water. Wash floor as usual. Empty bucket and fill with water and an additional 1 cup of white vinegar. Rinse floors with vinegar water as the final rinse and allow to dry to a shine.

Furniture and Wood Cleaning

Furniture Polish

Use this unique, old-time cleaning trick to restore natural wood to its original luster. Again, always testing a small spot before overall application to the wood.

In a small bowl, combine 1/8 cup of white vinegar with 1/4 cup linseed oil and 1/8 cup whiskey. Use this to wipe and polish wood furniture with a clean, soft cloth. Allow alcohol to evaporate as the solution air dries.

Furniture Polish for General Cleaning

Combine together 3/4 cup white vinegar with 1/4 cup lemon oil. Store this mixture in a jar with a tight-fitting lid for future use. Use as needed to polish wood furniture by wiping to a shine with a soft, clean cloth.

Furniture Polish and Cleaner

Mix together 1/2 cup each of white vinegar and olive oil. No need to use expensive olive oil for this; a general, all-purpose olive oil will do the trick just fine. Pour combined ingredients into a glass jar and seal with a tight fitting lid.

When ready to clean, use a clean cloth or rag to wipe solution onto wood furniture and buff dry.

Furniture with Waxes Surfaces

The key to washing furniture with waxed surfaces is to use cool water instead of warm. Warm water softens the wax coating, making it easier for tiny dirt particles and dust to become embedded in the wax, dulling its shine.

Add 1/2 cup of white vinegar to a bucket of cool water. Wash down waxed surfaces with a clean rag soaked in vinegar solution, or a damp mop. Dry smaller surfaces with a clean cloth, and allow wax flooring to air dry.

Wood Cleaning

Combine 1 teaspoon of white vinegar with 1 cup of warm water. Carefully wash wood surfaces to prevent haze build up common with commercial cleaners. Buff dry in a circular motion until completely dry and clean.

This method can also be used for larger cleaning areas, such as flooring. Just increase the amounts proportionally, and be careful not to saturate wood floors. Begin in one small area, treating each section separately until entire floor area is finished. Allow to air dry, taking care not to walk on sections until fully buffed and dry.

Wood Paneling

Mix together 1 tablespoon white vinegar with 1 tablespoon olive oil and 1 cup warm water in a small bowl. Using a clean cloth, wipe down wood paneling to perk up appearance and restore it to its natural beauty.

Wood Scratches

This simple solution can help repair gently scratches to wood furniture and flooring. Be sure to work lightly and gradually build in strength to reach your desired shade.

Combine 2 tablespoons of white vinegar with 2 tablespoons of iodine in a small dish. You will use this as your base for filling in and repairing scratches to wood. Using an artist's brush, carefully paint mixture deep into scratches and allow to air dry. For light colored scratches, add a little more vinegar to dilute the consistency. For dark colored scratches, add a little more iodine to darken and deepen the consistency.

Stainless in the Kitchen

Stainless Steel

Vinegar is a natural choice for cleaning and polishing stainless steel in the kitchen and elsewhere around the home.

Dampen a cleaning cloth with white vinegar and dip into 1 or 2 tablespoons of baking soda to coat. Gently rub onto stainless steel in a circular motion. Rinse with clean water and buff with dry side of a cloth until shiny clean.

Stainless Steel Appliances

Stainless steel appliances are a magnet for fingerprints. Dampen a soft cloth with undiluted white vinegar and wipe down the stainless steel portions of appliances. Polish dry without rinsing.

Stainless Steel Sinks

Use this formula to not only clean grime from stainless steel sinks, but to also remove rust stains from around the drain area.

Pour 1 teaspoon of salt over rust-stained spot in the sink drain. Drizzle about 1 tablespoon of white vinegar over salt and rub clean with a paper towel or cleaning cloth. When finished, use additional white vinegar to clean and polish the remainder of the sink area.

Laundry

Alpaca Fabric

After washing alpaca fabric as normal, rinse fabric in clean water to which 1 tablespoon of white vinegar has been added to keep it like new.

Angora

After normal method of washing, rinse angora in a basic of clean water with 2 tablespoons of white vinegar added. Gently remove any excess water, without wringing, and lay flat to dry.

Cigarette or Cigar Odor Removal

Cigarette and cigar odor can ruin fabrics fast. After washing clothing, hang odored garment above bathtub. Pour 3 cups of white vinegar into tub with very hot water and allow steam to rid clothing of smoke. Repeat the process, if necessary.

Clean and Whiten

Add 1/2 cup of undiluted white vinegar to the washing machine's wash cycle to clean and whiten clothing. Adding vinegar will also help kill the growth of fungus and inhibit mold. Run through the machine's rinse cycle as usual, and dry.

Cotton

Add 3/4 cup of white vinegar to laundry washing machine's final rinse cycle. Run as normal for softer cotton clothing. Great for cotton blankets and sheets, too.

Diapers

This is a wonderful solution for use in washing and disinfecting baby's cloth diapers. Vinegar will help disinfect, as well as discourage irritating diaper rashes on baby's delicate bottom.

Add 3/4 cup white vinegar to final rinse water for diapers (cloth diapers should always be rinsed twice). Fabric softeners should not be added to baby's diaper rinse water. These harsher chemical softeners may irritate baby's fragile skin and make cloth diapers less absorbent.

Fabric Softener, Gentler

Use this for scent-free laundry. Excellent for people who are allergic to chemical softeners.

Add 1/3 cup white vinegar to laundry's final rinse cycle, and then dry as usual.

Fabric Softener, Scent-Free

Combine 1/3 cup white vinegar with 1/3 cup baking soda in a cup. Add this mixture to final rinse water for soft, scent-free laundry every time.

Fabric Softener, Scented

Combine 1/2 cup apple cider vinegar with 1/3 cup baking soda in a small bowl or cup. Add this to final rinse water for a fresh, scented softener.

Leather Cleaning

Bring 1/2 cup white vinegar to a boil in a small saucepan. Add 2 or 3 vitamin E capsules and allow the capsules to dissolve completely. Remove from stovetop and add 1/2 cup olive oil, stirring until all ingredients are well blended. Cool solution and use to clean leather coats and boots.

Leather Polish

Combine 1/3 cup of white vinegar with 2/3 cup linseed oil and 1/3 cup clean water in a small bowl or tub. Apply to leather with a soft cloth. Using a second, clean cloth, buff to a high shine, removing any excess polish and you buff.

Leather Saddles and Boots

Work beeswax into 1/4 cup of white vinegar which has been slightly heated warm on the stovetop. Add a few drops of liquid soap and oil. Continue heating until all ingredients are soft and mixed together, then cool to room temperature. Use this clean horse saddles and cowboy boots.

Leather Shoes

Combine 1 tablespoon of white vinegar, 1 tablespoon rubbing alcohol, 1 teaspoon vegetable oil and 3 or 4 drops of your favorite liquid soap in a small bowl. Using a clean, soft cloth, gently wipe solution onto leather area of shoes. Using a second clean cloth, buff until leather shoes have reached a high shine. Be sure not to leave on any excess mixture that will build up and dull the shine of the leather.

Leather Shoes, Patent

Moisten a paper towel with undiluted white vinegar and gently rub into clean patent leather shoes. Using a second paper towel, finish by rubbing a slight amount, around 1 teaspoonful, of petroleum jelly into leather shoes and buff to a beautiful shine.

Lint Trap

Hard water can cause mineral buildup on washing machine and dryer lint traps. Use this solution to occasionally clean the trap.

Soak link trap in undiluted white vinegar for 2 hours. Brush away all mineral deposits clean with a cleaning brush. Rinse with clean water and replace. For heavily built-up deposits, this may need to be repeated a second time.

Musty Smell from Bedding or Drapes

Saturate cloth or hand towel with undiluted apple cider vinegar and wring out excess moisture. Place musty bedding in clothes dryer along with vinegared cloth. Set clothes dryer setting to "Air Dry" and run for 10 to 15 minutes, allowing vinegared cloth to soak up musty odors. Repeat, if necessary, or hang outside to complete drying.

Natural Red Dye Coloring

This solution allows you make your very own natural red dye for fabrics.

Wash 1 pound of beets and place them in a saucepan; cover with 1 quart of cool water. Simmer beets until they become tender, then remove skins. Chop beets and return to same water in which they were cooked. Allow beets to set for 2 hours. Strain off and save red liquid and combine with 1/2 cup of vinegar to achieve a beautiful, red fabric dye. After dying clothes or fabrics, always finish by drying in the dryer to "set" the color permanently.

Panty Hose Revitalizer

This works wonders on stretched out panty hose. In a small bowl or clean sink basin, combine 1/4 cup white vinegar with 1 quart of warm water. Soak panty hose for 5 minutes. Remove and gently squeeze out any excess moisture, being careful not to wring hose. Blot with a towel. Allow hose to air dry, spread out flat on a towel to help soak up water.

Pretreater

Pour 1 tablespoon white vinegar, 2 tablespoons ammonia and 1 tablespoon liquid laundry detergent into a spray bottle. Mix together by gently swirling. Add 2 tablespoons baking soda. When the reaction stops foaming, add cool water to within an inch of the top of the bottle. Use as a pretreater for hard to clean areas and clothing stains.

This should be stored indefinitely in the spray bottle, as the ingredients may damage the pump over time.

Removing/Adding Hems to Clothing

Dampen letdown hems with undiluted white vinegar prior to ironing to eliminate creases. To add creases to fabric or hems, again dampen with vinegar and iron in a new crease.

Removing Clothing Manufacturing Chemicals

Many people find themselves allergic to manufacturing dyes and chemicals found in new clothing. Use this solution to remove the chemicals prior to wearing for the first time.

Add 1/4 cup white vinegar to laundry's wash cycle when washing clothes for the first time. Run though wash and rinse cycle as usual.

Rinse

These ready-to-go, presoaked cloths are easy to add to the final rinse cycle of your laundry. They not only save measuring each time you do laundry, but keep vinegar from coming into direct contact with delicate fabrics.

Soak new or clean washcloths in undiluted white vinegar until fully saturated. Place cloths, one on top of another, in small plastic container or zipping plastic bag. Toss in one of these pretreated cloths into final rinse cycle of your washing machine each time you do laundry.

Saddle Soap

Warm 1/4 cup beeswax slowly over medium heat, and add 1/4 cup white vinegar. Add 1/8 cup liquid soap along with 1/8 cup linseed oil and stir together until incorporated. Keep moisture warm until it blends into a smooth texture. Remove from heat and cool until it reaches a solid state. When ready to use, rub saddle soap into leather, then buff to a high shine with a soft, clean cloth.

Setting Fabric Dyes

Use this formula to help "set" fabric dyes after coloring.

Fill bucket or sink with cold water. Add 1 cup white vinegar and 1 teaspoonful of salt. Soak newly dyed fabric in solution for 1 hour. Rinse in cold water to complete setting the dye.

Silks

Add 2 tablespoons of undiluted white vinegar to final rinse cycle and run as usual to keep silks like new. Do not rinse vinegar out.

Stain Removal

Combine together 3 tablespoons white vinegar with 3 tablespoons milk. Pour directly onto stain and gently rub fabric together. Allow to set for 5 minutes, then was as usual.

Stain Removal of Coffee and Tea Stains (dry)

This solution works best on coffee and tea stains that have already dried.

Soak stain in undiluted white vinegar for 30 minutes. Wash as normal to finish removing stain. If stain does not come out completely, repeat the process again before drying.

Stain Removal of Coffee and Tea Stains (wet)

This solution works best if stains are caught right away, before solution has a chance to dry.

Blot out as much coffee or tea as possible with a paper towel. Rinse in cool water, and wring out slightly. Pour white vinegar directly onto stain. Wash in lukewarm, soapy water to remove stain. Rinse as usual.

Stain Removal of Coffee and Tea that are Stubborn

For more stubborn coffee and tea stains that have still left a residue, try this solution. Wet stained area with white vinegar. Sprinkle about 1 teaspoon of salt directly onto dampened stain and set garment in bright sunlight for at least 1 hour. Wash and dry garment as usual. For very tough stains, you may want to repeat the process a second time.

Stain Removal of Inks

Soak ink stain in milk for one hour. Combine 1 tablespoon each of white vinegar and cornstarch, forming a thick paste. Cover the stain with paste and gently rub into cloth. Leave stain until paste dries, then wash away stain in your normal wash cycle.

Stain Removal of Iron Scorch Marks

Dampen a clean cloth with white vinegar. Blot vinegar onto scorched area of garment and allow to set for 5 minutes. If stain remains, repeat process again. If after 2 attempts scorching still remains, sprinkle a little salt over remoistened scorch and allow to set for 5 minutes. Now wash garment like usual in your normal wash cycle.

Stain Removal on Permanent Press

Wet stain with white vinegar and allow to set for 3 to 5 minutes. Wash in cool water and a clean rinse cycle.

Stain Removal of Perspiration Stains

Combine 1/4 cup white vinegar in 2 gallons of clean water; pour into a clean sink. Soak perspiration-stained clothing in this solution overnight. In the morning, wash as usual for full removal of stain.

Stain Removal of Rust Stains

Pour 1 tablespoon of white vinegar directly over rust stain, making sure to use enough vinegar to cover stain entirely. Sprinkle salt over dampened stain. Set outside in the bright sun for at least an hour to dry. Rinse out salt and reapply until stain disappears completely, Wash and rinse as usual.

Stain Removal of Wine

Blot undiluted white vinegar onto a wine stain. Stain should begin to dissipate and fade immediately. Wash as usual.

Stain Removal of Stubborn Wine

This is a strong formula for removing tough wine stains. Be careful to work gently into delicate fabrics. Blot up as much wine as possible from fabric. Saturate stain with 1 tablespoon of white vinegar and 3 tablespoons of water. While stain is still wet with vinegar solution, gently rub salt into stain. Set in sunlight to dry completely, then wash as usual.

Static Cling

Add 1/4 cup of white vinegar to laundry's final rinse cycle to eliminate static cling and reduce lint build up.

Straw Hats

Straw hats can become worn out and misshapen overtime. Try this formula to breathe new life into an old straw hat.

Pour 1/2 cup salt into a bucket of warm water and dissolve completely. Submerge straw hat in salt water solution. Once straw is slightly softened, remove from salt water and wipe away any stains with a clean cloth. For tough stains, add 1 or 2 drops of liquid detergent to a sponge and continue cleaning. Push and mold straw hat back into its original shape.

Pour 1 teaspoon of white vinegar into a spray bottle along with 1 cup of water. Once hat is in desired shape, spray hat with a fine mist of vinegar solution. Allow to air dry, but do not place in direct sunlight while drying.

Wool Sweaters

Add 1 cup white vinegar to laundry machine's final rinse cycle and run as normal. Wool sweaters will come out fluffy and new after this final vinegar rinse.

Nursery

Baby Bottle Nipples

In a clean pan, add 1 teaspoon white vinegar to 2 cups of water. Drop in baby bottle nipples and bring to a boil over medium heat. Allow to continue boiling for several minutes. This will not only clean and sterilize the nipples, but also keep them from developing a sour taste over time.

High Chair Cleaning

Set high chair in the shower and spray with full strength white vinegar. Allow to set for 5 to 10 minutes. Turn shower on with warm water and spray high chair for 3 minutes. Wipe food and grime off chair. Give a final rinse and wipe dry.

Odors

This is a great, non-invasive method for eliminating odor from baby's nursery.

Take a clean towel that has just been washed, but still damp, from the washing machine. Spray damp towel with vinegar and hang over door in baby's room. As towel dries, it will work to control odors and add clean moisture to the room.

Play Clay for Children

Here is a fun, non-toxic recipe for play clay that is completely natural and safe for children to use. Combine 1 teaspoon of white vinegar, 1 cup flour, 1/2 cup salt, 1 cup water and 1 tablespoon oil in a saucepan over medium heat. Stir continually until it forms into a ball. Remove from heat and allow to cool. Knead clay ball until smooth. Add a few drops of your preferred color of food coloring, if desired. Store in a tightly sealed container or wrapped in plastic wrap in the refrigerator when not in use.

Toys

In a small bowl, combine 1/4 cup white vinegar with 1 cup clean water. Use this solution to wipe down baby toys, plastic dolls and building blocks to keep play area clear of germs.

Toys

Combine 1/4 cup white vinegar and a few drops of dish detergent in 1 quart of hot water. Use to regularly wash down baby's playthings, including crib slats and bars. Rinse well and pat dry.

Office

Books

Combine 1 tablespoon white vinegar with 2 cups water in a spray bottle. Using a fine mist spray, spray a soft cloth with this weak vinegar solution. Use cloth to wipe books and dry immediately.

Bookshelves

Add 2 cups white vinegar to a bucket of warm water; add a few drops of your favorite dish detergent. Using a rag or sponge, wipe down bookshelves, being certain to get into corners and crevices to remove dust, dirt and odors.

Construction Paper Stains

Colored construction paper, when it becomes wet, can leave colored stains on desks and other furniture. Try this formula for simple and thorough removal. Combine 1/4 cup white vinegar and 1/4 cup water together. Use paper towels to blot up and clean wet construction paper stains.

Correction Fluid Stains

Dab area of furniture or cushion that has come into contact with correction fluid. Gently wipe with a paper towel to clean. If spot is persistent, slightly saturate stain with vinegar and blot away.

Super Glue on Fingers

Fill a small bowl with undiluted white vinegar. Soak affected fingers for several minutes. Peel away stuck glue.

Around the House

Air Freshener

Combine 1 tablespoon white vinegar with 1 teaspoon baking soda and 2 cups of water in a plastic spray bottle. Spray into the air in rooms needing a freshening up. Instead of just masking the odor, vinegar works to eliminate and neutralize the odor itself.

All-Purpose Cleaner

This is a wonderful, all-purpose cleaning solution to have on hand for many cleaning jobs around the house. Combine 1/4 cup white vinegar with 2 cups water and 3 tablespoons of liquid detergent in a plastic spray bottle. Use around the house for every day household cleaning. It is a great cleaner for high dust areas, like banisters and window baseboards, too.

Ceilings

Combine 1/2 cup white vinegar with 1 tablespoon of dish detergent in a bucket of warm water. In sections, use sponge or cloth to wash. Dry each section before you begin a new one. A new paint roller brush on an extended broom handle works well for this, too.

Room Deodorizer

Heat 1 cup apple cider vinegar and 1/4 cup water on stovetop until hot. Remove from heat and pour into a heat-safe bowl. Sprinkle 1 tablespoon cinnamon on top of vinegar solution. Place bowl on a low table in room to be freshened.

Painted Surfaces

Mix together 1/4 cup white vinegar with 1 tablespoon cornstarch and 2 cups of hot water in a bowl or storage cup. Wipe or spray solution onto painted surface. Immediately dry with a cloth. Do not allow liquid to soak into paint.

Painted Concrete Walls and Floors Preparation

This solution will help prepare concrete walls and floors for painting, cutting down on future peeling. Brush or paint concrete walls or floors with undiluted white vinegar as a preparation for painting. Allow to air dry thoroughly before applying paint.

Odor-Free Painting

Fill 3 small bowls with 1 cup white vinegar in each bowl. Place around room being painted to help absorb fresh paint odors while painting.

Paint Removal from Old Wood Windows

Combine 1/2 cup white vinegar with 1/2 cup liquid dish detergent and blend thoroughly. Use a paintbrush to brush vinegar mixture onto wood that needs paint to be removed. Soak for 10 minutes, then begin to carefully scrape away old paint with a razor scraper.

Walls

In a bucket, combine 1 cup white vinegar with warm water. Using a clean rag, wipe walls and allow to air dry. For markings on wall that do not seem to wipe away, try a quick rub with undiluted vinegar. Fill bucket wit warm rinse water. Add another cup of vinegar. With a clean cloth, use this solution to rinse walls clean.

Wallpaper Stripping

Combine 1 cup white vinegar with 1 tablespoon liquid detergent in a spray bottle. Wet wallpaper surface with vinegar solution and allow to set for 5 minutes. Gently remove wallpaper with scraper, adding more solution as you go. For difficult jobs, try "etching" wallpaper first with a scoring tool. Then wet wallpaper with solution and allow to set for another 5 minutes. Wallpaper should now peel or scrape free.

Window Cleaner, Streak Free

Mix all ingredients together in a plastic spray bottle. Spray onto windows and mirrors. Wipe immediately with a soft cloth or paper towel.

Window Cleaner, Deep Cleaning

In a small bowl, combine 1/4 cup white vinegar with 1/4 cup

cornstarch and dab thick solution onto dirty windows. Allow this paste to dry into a chalky film. Rub off with a soft cloth using a circular motion until completely clean.

Window Cleaning Cloths

Combine 1/4 cup white vinegar with 1/2 teaspoon liquid dish soap and 2 cups of water. Using a clean cloth, dip into mixture and wring out. Store damp coated cloth in a glass jar with tight fitting lid. Wipe spots from windows and mirrors, as needed.

Window Drapes

This is a wonderful solution to freshen up drapery from existing odors and add a new freshness to the room. Be sure drapes are free of heavy dust before wetting. Dust can be eliminated with tools from your vacuum cleaner.

In a plastic spray bottle, combine 2 cups of warm water with 1 tablespoon white vinegar and shake gently to combine. Spritz each drapery panel and moisten drapes completely, paying particular attention to add a little extra solution to any heavily wrinkled areas.

Allow to air dry, still hanging on the windows. Drapes will smell fresher, and most of all, the wrinkles will disappear.

Window Drapes and Fiberglass

Fiberglass drapes demand special attention when getting cleaned. Try this formula to clean fiberglass drapes, while still keeping their delicate integrity.

Hang drapes firmly on a clothesline and spray gently with a hose, fully wetting the drapes. Fill plastic spray bottle with 2 cups of water with 1 tablespoon white vinegar. Spray drapes with vinegar solution and allow to dry on clothesline for ultimate freshness.

Window Shutters and Louvered Doors

Fill a spray bottle with undiluted white vinegar. Wrap a soft, clean cloth around a paint stirring stick or ruler. Spray cloth with vinegar and run it over, beneath and between each louver to get rid of dust and built up grime.

Miscellaneous

Ash Trays

Combine 1/8 white vinegar with 1/8 cup hot water. Fill ashtray with this mixture and allow to set overnight to get rid of lingering smoke odors.

Aquariums

This solution is excellent for clearing the outside glass of a fish aquarium. However, it should never be used to clean the inside of the tank, as the vinegar could be toxic to fish. Always spray vinegar onto cloth, and not directly on aquarium glass. Tiny droplets may get into the aquarium water and upset the delicate pH balance, possibly harming the fish.

Mix a teaspoon white vinegar and 1 cup water and pour into a spray bottle. Spray soft cloth with vinegar solution and wipe clean aquarium exterior. Buff dry. If aquarium exterior is extremely dirty, use undiluted vinegar and wipe clean.

Ballpoint Pen Stains

Wet area stained with ballpoint pen with undiluted white vinegar. You can do this by drizzling vinegar over the area and allow to penetrate the stained area of cloth. For areas that are vertical, like walls, soak a clean cloth in vinegar and place against stain. Allow to soak in for 10 minutes. Blot up with a clean cloth. Repeat, if necessary. Thoroughly dry, when finished.

Chewing Gum

Try this solution for chewing gum that gets stuck on just about anything, including fabrics.

Soak chewing gum in undiluted white vinegar until it begins to dissolve. If gum will not dissolve, repeat above steps with heated vinegar.

Eyeglasses

Drench cotton ball or soft cloth with white vinegar. Wipe eyeglasses clean and allow to air dry for streak-free cleaning.

Fireplace Ashes

This vinegar water solution keeps ashes from flying around the room and helps neutralize alkali in the ash.

Fill a spray bottle with 2 tablespoons of white vinegar and 2 cups of water. Before scooping out ashes, spray them down with a coating of vinegar and water solution. Now scoop out wet ashes (this will help keep them from flying al over the room). Continue to spray as you clean to keep dust and ask particles to a minimum. When finished scooping out ashes, use remaining vinegar solution to thoroughly clean fireplace if finished using for the season.

Garbage Cans

Pour a half gallon of water in an empty garbage can and add 1 cup of white vinegar. Swirl around bottom and edges of can and then place in direct sunlight. As it dries, it will not only disinfect, but also rid can of lingering garbage odors.

Glass or Beaded Jewelry

Combine 1 quart of water with 1 teaspoon of liquid detergent. Dip strand of beads into water. Remove immediately and dip into second bowl of warm water with 1 tablespoon of vinegar to rinse clean. Blot dry with a paper towel and complete drying with hair dryer on lowest setting.

Hairbrushes

Mix 1/2 cup white vinegar, 2 cups hot water and 2 or 3 cups of liquid dish soap. Completely immerse hairbrushes in vinegar solution and allow to soak for 30 minutes. Rub hairbrushes together to clean and rinse thoroughly. Allow to air dry.

Hairbrushes, Combs and Rollers

Keeping hairbrushes, combs and rollers clean is essential to beautiful hair. Combine 1 cup white vinegar and 1 quart of warm water in a large bowl or sink. Place brushes, combs and rollers in vinegar water and allow to soak for one hour. Remove and brush away any lingering build up with old toothbrush to which a few drops of liquid detergent has been added. Rinse with clean, clear water.

Refill sink basin with warm water and add 1/4 cup additional white vinegar. Rinse brushes and combs clean one last time. Allow to air dry on a towel.

Humidifiers

Add two tablespoons of white vinegar to water in a humidifier to eliminate odors in your home as it humidifies. Vinegar also discourages bacteria and mold growth in the humidifier's water receptacle.

Lamp Shades

Place 2 cups of white vinegar and 3 tablespoons liquid detergent in a bucket of hot water. Take an old lamp shade and immerse one corner of the shade in tube of water and move it around vigorously to clean. Take shade out, turn to a different corner, and repeat until entire shade has been cleaned. Remove shade from water and empty tub. Refill tub with clean water and add another cup of vinegar. Repeat same clean and shake motion to now rinse lampshade. Allow to air dry.

Moth Repellent

Mix 1/2 cup white vinegar with 1/4 cup lavender in a small jar. Leave jar open in moth-ridden areas of the house. Also saturate small cloths or sachets with this solution, and place in areas you wish to rid of moths.

Moth Repellent

Heat 2 cups white vinegar on stovetop and add 1/2 cup torn lavender leaves. Simmer for 10 minutes and remove from heat. Allow to cool completely. Pour into a jar with a tight-fitting lid. Allow to steep for 10 days. Use to wipe down walls and plastic storage bins in clothes closet to drive away moths.

Silk House Plants

In a small bowl, combine 1/4 cup white vinegar with 1 quart of warm water. Use a paper towel or cleaning rag to dab in solution and wipe dust and dirt from silk and plastic house plants. Allow to air dry. You can also pour this solution into a plastic spray bottle and use to spray silk plants to keep dust from forming in the first place.

Sticker or Decal Removal

Wet a cotton ball or paper towel with white vinegar. Saturate sticker or decal with vinegar. Soak until sticker can be removed. Repeat if necessary, until sticker and glue residue comes free. For stickers that will not come loose, gently scratch the top layer off, or scratch grooves into the paper. Then, repeat steps above, allowing to soak until sticker breaks free.

Urine Stained Mattress

This mixture will not only remove unsightly urine stains from mattresses, but also the unpleasant odor that accompanies it.

Spray urine-stained area of mattress with white vinegar, and allow to set for 3 to 5 minutes. Use a cloth or paper towel to blot dry. You may need to repeat process again until entire stain comes clean.

Wet Dry Vac

Wet Dry Vacs tend to smell musty after time. Try using this formula periodically to freshen vac and extend the life of the appliance.

Mix 2 cups white vinegar with 2 quarts warm water. Suck up solution in vac and allow to set for 5 minutes. Empty machine and wipe out inside of vac. Allow vac to air dry completely before putting it back together for storage.

Septic System

First, clean drains throughout the house by pouring 1/2 cup baking soda down drain, and follow with 1/2 cup white vinegar. Allow each drain to rest with baking soda and vinegar solution for 10 minutes. Then, run hot water down the drain to rinse clean.

Next, pour 1 package of dry yeast and 2/3 cup brown sugar into toilet and flush the tank twice.

Schedule this periodic preventative maintenance by putting it on your calendar. Doing this routine monthly will not only keep drains running clean, but also help the septic system to run efficiently for many years.

Chapter Five
Out and About

B enefits of vinegar have been long proven throughout the ages. They are well known in both medicinal and cleaning circles, as well as its use as an effective health and beauty product. But one aspect of vinegar that is sometimes overlooked is its use in the field of agriculture.

Why Vinegar in Agriculture?

As we have previously discussed, vinegar is all-natural, meaning it comes from nature itself without the addition of harmful chemicals. Its very makeup is a rich combination of vitamins, minerals and essential nutrients not commonly found together. It also possesses a storehouse of properties that make it uniquely effective in farming and gardening:

- Antifungal properties that help eliminate harmful fungus from plants
- Antibiotic elements which can be used to stave off disease in farm animals and pets
- Antimicrobial traits which can kill and stop the spread and growth of dangerous microorganisms
- Antiseptics that can help heal injury to a host of animals
- Anti-inflammatory characteristics which are also beneficial to farming animals as well as household pets
- The ability to help balance pH levels in the soil
- Makes a potent insecticide that is effective for pest control but completely safe for human consumption
- Improves germination among difficult to sprout seed types
- Acts as an effective solution against slugs, snails and other

garden infestations
- Its potent aroma can help deter unwanted garden rodents

This chapter will cover some of the best, as well as least known, vinegar applications for gardening, farming and even household pet uses. Some of these helps date back generations and have been passed down from family to family. One of the main benefits of using vinegar in the place of more common gardening products is not only vinegar's effectiveness, but also lack of toxicity which might otherwise be harmful for consumption or damage soil.

Enjoy using these tips for more beautiful gardens, robust crops and healthier livestock.

Cut Flowers
Combine 1 tablespoon white vinegar with 2 cups water and 2 tablespoons sugar in a vase. Take a group of flowers and, below some cool running water, cut stems at an angle. Place in vinegar and sugar water for beautiful, long lasting blooms.

Birdbaths
This solution is great for controlling growth of fungus and bacteria in outdoor birdbaths. Add 2 tablespoons white vinegar to outdoor birdbath water every time you refill the bath to keep water bacteria free, and fresh for drinking and bathing.

Fruit Flies
Pour 1 cup of apple cider vinegar into a glass mason jar and add a few drops of liquid detergent. Poke a few tiny holes in the plastic wrap with a toothpick and place over the mouth of the glass jar. Secure in place with a rubber band and place on kitchen counter near fruit.

Fruit flies will be attracted to the apple cider vinegar and fall into the liquid. The liquid detergent acts as a barrier in the water and fruit flies will be unable to get back out.

Hummingbird Feeders

Use white vinegar to clean and disinfect an empty hummingbird feeder. Rinse and wipe dry before using.

Soaps and detergents can be toxic to delicate birds, but because vinegar is natural, it makes the perfect cleaning solution that is powerful enough to disinfect, but delicate enough not to harm birds.

Outdoor Water Fountains

Add 1/2 to 1 cup of white vinegar to outdoor water fountains to keep fountain pumps running clean, disinfect from bacteria and discourage mold or moss growth.

Rusty Tools

Using liberal amounts of white vinegar, wash down rusty garden tools allowing the rusted areas to become completely soaked in vinegar. Allow to set for 10 minutes and wipe away rust.

Cats in the Garden

Outdoor cats in the sandbox or garden can pose a real problem. To keep them away without harm, sprinkle white vinegar in a child's sandbox or around the garden to prevent roaming cats from using the area as their own personal litter box.

Balancing Soil pH Levels

Proper pH levels in the soil is essential to good gardening and farming. And vinegar is the natural choice. Pour white vinegar into a bucket of clean water. Pour in a circle around acid-loving plants, such as azaleas, blueberries, marigolds and radishes to balance soil's pH level and help plants thrive.

Clay Flowerpots

Mineral deposits not only make the clay pots appear unsightly, but can also interfere with the way clay pots breathe and absorb water. To clean and restore, simply dip a scrub brush into white vinegar and scrub the outside of the pots. If the pot is empty, also clean the inside of the pot. Use fresh water to rinse clean.

Cucumber and Melon Plants

Combine 2 cups white vinegar with 1/4 cup oregano leaves and allow to set for at least 15 minutes to incorporate. Wet ground area around cucumber or melon plants every week to keep bugs from eating and infesting plants.

Fungus

Combine 1 tablespoon vinegar with 1 cup chamomile tea and spray directly onto plants to safely eliminate plant fungus.

Herbicide

Try this mixture on hard-to-kill vegetation infiltrating gardens and walk paths. It can also be used to kill any unwanted grass growing in the cracks of driveways, paths and sidewalks.

Combine 2 quarts white vinegar and 1/3 cup salt in a bowl and stir until salt is completely dissolved. Pour vinegar salt mixture into a plastic spray bottle and add 1 tablespoon liquid dish detergent and 1 teaspoon cayenne pepper. Use this solution directly on any vegetation you want to kill, paying particular attention to completely soaking the plant's leaves.

Herbicide Spray

Combine 2 cups white vinegar in a spray bottle with 1/4 cup salt, making sure to completely dissolve salt before attempting to use sprayer. Spray solution on unwanted grass or weed areas and allow to completely saturate.

Problem Insects

Combine 1/4 cup white vinegar, 3/4 cup water and a few drops of liquid detergent in a spray bottle. Use to spray tender garden plants that are being overtaken by troublesome insects.

Nasturtium Germination

Some seeds can use a little help with the germination process. Try this trick for quicker germination and stronger seeds. Combine 1/8 teaspoon white vinegar with 2 cups of water in a bowl and soak nasturtium seeds overnight before planting. The following morning, be sure and plant seeds while they are still damp for best and quickest growth.

Okra

Mix 1/8 teaspoon white vinegar with 1 and 1/2 cups water in a bowl. Soak okra seeds overnight before planting for faster growth.

Paths and Stones

Combine 1/2 cup white vinegar with 1 tablespoon fresh thyme. Sprinkle or spray onto garden paths and stepping stones as a wonderful, natural pest repellent. This concoction will also help keep mold and mildew from forming on stones.

Tomatoes

Mix together 1 cup white vinegar with 1/4 cup chopped basil leaves and allow to set for at least 15 minutes before using. Soak ground beneath tomato plants to keep harmful insects away.

Varmints

Soak spare rags in white vinegar and place around garden as a deterrent for varmints.

Varmint Solutions

Soak cotton balls in apple cider vinegar and place strategically around garden. The vinegar will not only keep varmints and insects at bay, but is also helpful for continuing to balance pH levels in the soil itself.

Garden Vegetables

Combine 2 cups white vinegar with 1/4 cup chopped sage and store in a plastic bottle. Sprinkle sage-vinegar solution around vegetable vines to keep plant eating insects away.

Insects

Ants in the Home

Fill a spray bottle with undiluted white vinegar. Use to spray cupboards and countertops to rid home of ants.

Ants around the Home

Pour white vinegar into a spray bottle and use to spray a defining barrier around home's entry points, such as windows and doors.

Fire Ant Hills

Saturate ant hills with undiluted white vinegar to get rid of the ants. May need to repeat, making sure vinegar is working its way down the hill.

Anthills

Pour undiluted white vinegar directly into an anthill opening to kill the hill.

Aphids

Combine 2 cups white vinegar and about 1 cup of shredded mint leaves; allow to set for 10 minutes. Wet a circle of ground around cabbage, brussels sprouts and cauliflower plants with this mint-vinegar mixture to keep aphids from dining on plants.

Fleas

Combine 2 cups white vinegar with 1/2 cup torn basil leaves and warm on the stovetop. Simmer for 20 minutes and then cool completely. Pour in a thick line along home's entry to doorways to prevent fleas from entering the house.

Flying Insects

Pour 1/4 cup white vinegar into a plastic spray bottle. Crush 2 bay leaves and add to vinegar. Spray down picnic table and outlying area to keep flies and other insects at bay.

Mosquitoes

Warm 2 cups white vinegar on stovetop and add 1/2 cup lavender flowers. Simmer for 10 minutes. Cool completely and pour into a bowl or jar. Sprinkle around yard to keep mosquitoes at bay.

Snails and Slugs

Combine 1/2 cup white vinegar with 1/2 cup water in a spray bottle and use directly on snails and slugs for elimination.

Livestock

Cattle

Add 2 tablespoons apple cider vinegar per gallon of water to troughs to help protect cattle and other livestock from illness.

Chickens

Add 1/4 teaspoon of white vinegar to chickens' water each day to help support better growth. It is also thought that chickens consuming vinegar tend to be more tender, and increases egg production.

Chicken Disinfectant

Fill a plastic spray bottle with white vinegar and use to clean and disinfect chicken coups.

Flies

Pour 1 cup white vinegar into 1 cup water and add to a spray bottle. Use to spray livestock to keep irritating flies away.

Horses

Use 1/2 cup white vinegar to sprinkle directly on hay as a preventative for kidney stones and colic in horses.

Pigs

Add 1 cup apple cider vinegar to a 20 gallon water tough for pigs.

Livestock Skin Conditions

Combine 2 quarts apple cider vinegar with 2 cups warm water and pour solution directly over livestock with skin rashes and itches. Allow the solution to soak into the affected area and air dry. The strong vinegar smell will evaporate as the vinegar itself dries.

Chapter Six
Pets are People, Too

Beloved pets are important and special members of the family. The bring joy, excitement and love to those around them, and as such are entitled to the same safe, natural benefits vinegar offers their human counterparts. Vinegar's same medicinal properties, disinfecting qualities and healing attributes provide a natural alternative for treating our loved pets.

What Can Vinegar Do for Pets?

Vinegar has as many uses for pets as it does for their owners. Not only can vinegar be used to disinfect cuts, scrapes and injured areas, but it can also be depended on as a treatment for illness and a preventative medicine. And while much of the uses for vinegar mirror that of human use, vinegar can also provide helps specific to pet needs:

- Behavior issues
- Fleas and ticks
- Fur, skin and coat issues
- Urine stains
- Pet odor

Keep in mind that pets respond to vinegar much in the same way as the rest of us. Some pets may enjoy the taste, others may not. What works for one pet may work even better for another. And do not be afraid to make adaptations based on each pet's needs.

Enjoy discovering ways that vinegar can be used everyday for healthy, happy pets.

Behavior Issues

This is a simple solution to help treat a pet's behavior issues easily, quickly and without harm.

Fill a plastic squirt gun with water leaving a small amount of room. Add 1 teaspoon white vinegar. When pet approaches a forbidden area or begins to engage in behavior (such as scratching or chewing), tell him a stern "No" and reinforce the words with a quick liquid reminder. Soon, simply picking up the squirt gun will ensure good behavior. Eventually, once the bad habit is broken, no reminder will be needed at all.

Pet Bowls and Dishes

Use this safe vinegar solution to clean and disinfect pets' food and water dishes. Because these surfaces remain damp throughout the day, they likely harbor harmful bacteria and mold that can be unhealthy for both pets and people. Using vinegar on pets' surfaces avoids the need to use harsher chemicals, such as chlorine-based bleach, that might be harmful to the animal.

Pour 1/4 cup of white vinegar into pet's food or water dish and fill the rest of the way to the top with water. Allow to soak for 20 minutes and wash as usual. Make this part of your weekly cleaning routine to disinfect.

Dog Itching and Scratching

Shampoo and rinse dog as usual. Combine 1/3 cup apple cider vinegar and 2 quarts warm water in a clean bucket and pour over dog as his final rinse. Do not rinse again. Dry dog as usual and coat will be shiny and soft, cutting down on itching and scratching.

Fleas on Pets

Combine 1 cup white vinegar and 1 tablespoon chopped rue in a small bowl. Rub this concentration into dog's hair to discourage the start, or get rid of, nasty fleas.

Flea Protection

Combine 1/2 cup white vinegar with 1/4 cup water and 1 tablespoon fennel, then pour into a spray bottle. Using this spray, thoroughly saturate areas where pets sleep or play. Allow to air dry.

Pet Fur

Add 1 teaspoonful apple cider vinegar to the dog or cat's water dish to keep their coats shiny and healthy.

Jellyfish Stings

Keep a bottle of white vinegar on hand when taking your dog on vacation to the ocean where jellyfish may be a problem. At first suspicion of a jellyfish sting, pour undiluted vinegar over the sting area to help dilute the poison.

Bothersome Shedding

Try this easy method of removing pet hair from carpet, furniture or clothing.

Turn an old tube sock inside out and slip it over your hand. Lightly spray sock with white vinegar that has been poured into a spray bottle. Use dampened sock to wipe down furniture, carpet or clothing to remove unwanted pet hair. Dampened sock may also be used to wipe down your pet directly, removing shedded hair and leaving fur shiny and beautiful.

Horse's Coat

Pour 1/8 cup apple cider vinegar into horse's water trough every day to help keep his coat shiny and healthy.

Illness Fighter

Add 1 teaspoonful of apple cider vinegar to pet's water dish to help boost immune system during an illness.

Long-Haired Cats

Combine together 3 tablespoons white vinegar with 1 quart warm water. After bathing cat, rinse long fur in this warm vinegar solution. Fur will shine and any mats will brush out easier.

Pet Odor

Pour 2 tablespoons white vinegar and 2 cups water into a spray bottle. Spray pet's coat daily to help eliminate odor. Keep a bottle full of this mixture on hand for daily odor control for all types of furry pets.

Skunk Spray

Pets always seem to find a way to encounter the wrong end of a skunk. When they do, try this trick to eliminate odor. Wet a clean towel with undiluted white vinegar and use it to rub down a dog or cat that has been sprayed with skunk spray. Allow the pet's fur to air dry, and repeat if necessary, a second time.

Ticks

Try using this solution before heading outdoors to protect your hunting dog from ticks. Combine undiluted white vinegar with about 1/2 cup chamomile flowers in a small bowl. Set aside to soak for 15 minutes, allowing the flowers to thoroughly incorporate into the vinegar. Wipe this aromatic mixture directly onto dog's coat to discourage ticks.

Pet Urine

If urine stains on carpet or flooring are still damp, blot up as much as possible with a paper towel. Using vinegar in a spray bottle, completely dampen area of urine stain. Sprinkle baking soda over dampened stain. Using a scrub brush, brush stained area in a circular motion. Allow to dry completely. When dry, vacuum up stain and any residue.

It is important to be sure area is completely dry before vacuuming. Vacuuming damp residue can clog and damage the appliance.

Urine

Blot up any excess urine with a paper towel. Spray white vinegar directly over entire urine area. Allow to soak in for 2 to 3 minutes and blot up vinegar liquid with another paper towel. Repeat, as necessary.

Chapter Seven
The Great Outdoors

Vinegar has more uses, both inside and outside the house, than most people can imagine. For every commercial cleaning product application, there is usually a more natural, vinegar counterpart that can do the job just as well — or even better!

In addition to the more well known uses for vinegar, it can also be used on a variety of outdoor scenarios from cleaning and degreasing the family barbeque grill to cleaning filthy and forgotten window screens. In fact, it is a fantastic use for rehabbing old properties and bringing them back to their original luster.

Why Vinegar?

Vinegar is comprised of multiple traits that make it one of the most versatile liquids available. But even as strong as vinegar is, it is still all-natural which makes it a safer choice to use in circumstances where toxic chemical alternatives are not an option. It is safe around children and pets, but still effective enough to be used as a potent weed killer. Its acidic nature makes it an excellent choice when you are looking for ways to cut through tough grease and stains, but still need to prevent "etching" of surfaces like fiberglass or chrome.

It is unparalleled in its disinfecting ability, as some of its less talked about uses cannot be overlooked. It is excellent for removing invasive vegetation, as well as balancing delicate pH levels in farming or gardening soil. It is highly acidic in nature and possesses an innate ability to neutralize even the most foul odors.

The same attributes that make vinegar a powerful degreaser,

also render it an effective choice for cleaning and revitalizing tools. Its uses are nearly limitless.

Make vinegar your go-to choice for just about everything under the sun:

- Barbeque grills
- Boats
- Campers
- Automobiles
- Fiberglass
- Cement
- Oil stains
- Weeds

Use this next chapter as a springboard for uses of your own!

Barbeque Grills

Remove soiled barbeque rack from grill and place it in a plastic garbage bag. Fill a spray bottle with 2 cups white vinegar, and use to spray down entire rack until wet. Tie the garbage bag in a loose knot to seal in the moisture and place back with rack inside in the warm sun. Leave to soak for about 4 hours.

Untie the bag (be careful not to rip it) and add about 2 tablespoons of liquid dish washing detergent and 2 quarts of hot water. Retie bag and allow to soak in the sun for an additional 2 hours. Open the bag and use a cleaning rag to easily wipe the rack clean.

Boat Stains and Discoloration

Aluminum boats are extremely sensitive to alkaline in the water, which can etch aluminum and cause discoloration. White vinegar is an excellent source to neutralize alkaline, making it easier to scrub away discoloration.

Using a towel saturated with white vinegar, wipe clean any stains or discoloration appearing on boat. For heavy stains, spray vinegar directly onto boat and let stand for about 15 minutes before cleaning. Rinse clean with clear water and wipe dry.

Camper and RV Fiberglass

Spray areas of fiberglass camper or RV with undiluted vinegar where hard water has left stains. Wipe down with cloth and dry completely.

For tough to clean stains, soak a paper towel in vinegar and "stick" on top of the stain for 5 minutes. Remove paper towel and wipe clean. Rinse and dry completely.

Easy Laundry Cleaning While Camping

No easy access to a laundry machine while you are on the road? Try this novel, but functional method for washing laundry while camping. Using this solution, a watertight container is used as a "washing machine" to launder clothing while you are driving. The motion of driving works to agitate laundry and clean clothing. You will arrive at your day's destination with clean clothes, ready to rinse fresh and air dry.

In a watertight container, add 1 cup white vinegar, 2 or 3 tablespoons of liquid laundry detergent and 5 gallons of clean water. Place dirty clothing in container and make certain to seal tightly. Secure in camper and proceed on day's drive. When you arrive at your destination, rinse with clean water and hang outside to dry.

Car Air Freshener

This is a great solution to make in advance and keep on hand for a quick and easy air freshener in cars. Trial-size spray bottles are perfect for this one.

Fill a fine mist spray bottle with undiluted apple cider vinegar. Gently mist the interior of your car for a fresh, clean smell anytime.

Ashtrays

Wipe out a dirty ashtray with wadded up newspaper or a paper towel that has been drenched in white vinegar. Allow to air dry. Vinegar will neutralize away any ashtray odor leaving your car smelling fresh and clean.

Bumper Sticker Removal

Completely saturate a cloth or small towel in white vinegar. Do not wring out. Wrap soaked vinegar cloth around bumper where decal is attached. Allow to set undisturbed for 45 minutes. Remove wet towel and pull off sticker. Repeat again, if necessary. You may wish to use soaked towel to further wipe off any residual glue once sticker has been removed.

Car Chrome

Wipe down car chrome with undiluted white vinegar. Buff dry to a high shine with a soft, clean cloth.

Chrome Rust Spots

Tear off a small piece of aluminum foil and dip it into white vinegar. Rub out small rust spots on chrome until they are completely gone. Rinse away debris and dry completely with a clean towel. Using a small amount of car wax, add a wax coating to the area that was rusted to protect chrome and prevent new rust spots from forming.

Car Interior Windows

Combine 1/2 cup white vinegar with 1/4 cup clean water. Use a paper towel or chamois to wipe fingerprints and smudges from interior car windows for a streak-free shine.

Windshield Washer Cleaning Fluid

This is an excellent windshield washer cleaner for a no-streak, no-freeze cleaner. In a small clean bucket, combine 6 cups water with 1 tablespoon liquid detergent. Add 1/2 cup white vinegar and 2 cups rubbing alcohol and be sure to combine well. Pour this into windshield washer reservoir.

Vinyl Interiors

Combine 1/2 cup white vinegar, 1 teaspoon liquid soap and 1/2 cup water in a small bowl. Wipe this onto vinyl surfaces with a clean, soft cloth. Rinse gently with clear water and buff dry.

Grass Growing in Driveway Cracks

Pour white vinegar directly into cracks in driveway or sidewalk where grass is growing between the blocks. Check back in a couple of days and repeat, if necessary.

Grass Growing Between Cracks and Paving Stones

Combine 2 cups white vinegar with 3 tablespoons salt in a spray bottle and swirl to completely dissolve salt (do not place sprayer on bottle until salt has been completely dissolved). Use this solution to spray onto unwanted grass growing from cracks in the driveway and sidewalk, or between paving stones. Be certain not to treat any grass you do not wish to be removed.

Brooms

Use this idea to give a second life to an old, about-to-be-discarded broomstick hidden away in the garage.

Using a sharp knife or scissors, carefully cut about a third of the length of the broom's very worn bristles off, cutting at a deep angle (leaving the short side about 1 inch in length and the longer side about 6 inches in length).

Add 1 cup apple cider vinegar to a bucket of hot water and soak the newly cut broom for about 15 minutes to soften the bristles. Remove broom and shake, getting rid of most of the excess vinegar liquid. Set broom outside in direct sunlight and allow to completely air dry. When completely dry, use this new angled broom to reach hard to clean floor corners.

Cement Garage Floor

This simple, but powerful, solution can help clean a dirty garage floor like new.

In a bucket, add 1 cup white vinegar to 1 gallon of water. Take a pile of shredded newspaper and pour vinegar solution over it. Toss the wet, shredded newspaper over the worst spots of the garage floor and allow to set for 5 to 10 minutes. Sweep garage floor with a push broom. Dust and debris will cling to the newspaper, while the white vinegar acts to help neutralize garage odors.

Cement Garage Floor Dirt

Simple grass clippings, saved from a recent mowing, will help clean dust and other debris from dirty garage floors.

Spread handfuls of grass clippings around garage floor. Sprinkle apple cider vinegar over the discarded clippings and allow to set for 10 minutes. Use additional apple cider vinegar if necessary, but it does not need to coat all the clipping entirely. Using a push broom, sweep the cement flooring clean. The resulting garage floor will not only be clean, but the apple cider vinegar also gives the entire garage a fresh smell.

Garage Floor Oil Stains

This solution is hard working to remove oil stains from a leaky car engine.

Soak up as much standing oil as possible with paper towels and discard. Sprinkle a heavy coat of powdered laundry detergent (1 to 2 cups) over oil stain and allow to absorb. Using a push broom, brush away oil that has now adhered itself to the detergent. Repeat, if necessary, until majority of the stain is removed.

Add 1 cup white vinegar to about 1/2 gallon water in a bucket, and pour over old stained area. Spray with a garden hose for final rinse.

Tough Garage Floor Oil Stains

This idea works to remove hard to clean oil stains, or stains that have left behind a residue.

Use paper towels to soak up as much oil as possible form garage flooring and discard. Pour a heavy coating of cat litter directly on top of oil stain. Allow it soak up oil for about 20 to 30 minutes. Use a push broom to push away oil-soaked cat litter and discard into a trash can.

Combine 1 cup white vinegar with 1/2 gallon water in a bucket and pour over the old stain. Spray with a garden hose to remove any residue. For very tough stains, you may want to repeat.

Old Paintbrushes

Pour 1 quart white vinegar into a large, heavy pot and add dirty paintbrushes. Bring to a boil. Cover pot and remove from stovetop and allow to rest for one hour. Place vinegar pot with brushes back on stovetop and bring once again to a gentle boil. Simmer for 20 minutes.

Rinse brushes well, working the softened paint out of the bristles with your fingers or a metal painter's comb. For extremely heavy paint encrustations, repeat the process a second time before allowing to air dry.

Garage Tools

Combine 1/4 cup white vinegar with 1 quart of water and use together to wipe away any mineral buildup on metal tools.

Luggage Odor

Do you store your luggage in the garage or another area where odor can build up? Simply wet a cloth with 1/4 cup white vinegar and wring out the excess. Place damp cloth in luggage and close, but do not zipper shut. Allow to set overnight to eliminate odor.

Plastic Picnic Coolers

Empty a plastic picnic cooler that has become dirty or musty and wipe out all the food crumbs and debris. Pour 1 cup white vinegar, 1 teaspoon liquid detergent and 1 gallon water into the cooler. Using a clean cloth, make sure solution soaks into all areas of the cooler, including inside the lid. Put lid back onto cooler and allow to set while you wipe down the outside of the cooler.

To clean the outside, combine a second cup of vinegar with 1 cup of water. Use a cloth to wipe down cooler's exterior. Open cooler and dump out all the contents. Wipe down the inside and rinse thoroughly. Dry entire cooler.

Window Screens

Combine 1 cup white vinegar with 1/2 gallon water in a bucket and use a sponge to clean dirty window screens. For screens with heavy buildup, pretreat prior to sponge cleaning by putting vinegar in a spray bottle and wetting screens literally first. Allow these screens to set for 10 minutes and then proceed to clean with a wet sponge.

Chapter Eight
Vinegar & Diet

A recent study from the Center for Disease Control's National Center for Health Statistics shows the obesity rate in the United States now stands at a whopping 39.9%. That is nearly 40% of the U.S. population that is considered obese, and doesn't include people that fall into the "overweight" category.

It is often said in health circles that you cannot out exercise a bad diet. Health and wellness does not necessarily equal input (calories taken in) versus output (calories expended during exercise). One can be underweight, but still not healthy. Likewise, someone can be holding onto a few extra pounds, but be more fit than someone weighing less.

The Problem with Diets

As a culture, too often we fall into "diet mode" when we find ourselves overweight. While dieting may shed unwanted pounds in the short term, it is more often than not inadequate in the long term. Soon after completing a diet, pounds begin to creep back on, and we find ourselves right back where we started, or worse yet, weighing more than when we began. The reason this happens is two fold.

First, when we restrict the intake of calories, our bodies naturally go into a self-defense mode and our metabolism is lowered. This means our bodies burn calories more slowly in order to hold onto them as long as possible. It is a natural defense mechanism to avoid starvation. So, calories are not burned at the rate they normally should be, which can make weight loss more difficult.

Second, most people, upon completion of a diet, revert to their former eating habits. And in most cases, those very same habits helped cause them to become overweight in the first place.

In both cases, the person dieting winds up in exactly the same position they originally found themselves in, but now feels discouraged and defeated.

Albert Einstein was quoted as saying, "Insanity is doing the same thing over and over, but expecting different results." Simply put, successful weight loss requires a new mindset.

Ongoing wellness and maintaining a healthy weight begins with prevention. That means avoiding bad habits, such as excessive drinking and drug use to being proactive in adding health-building foods into your daily diet. And one of the very best foods to consider for both heathy living and weight loss is apple cider vinegar.

Many people swear to have success in shedding extra pounds and maintaining a healthy weight through the use of apple cider vinegar. The general thought behind this is that apple cider vinegar, when taken daily with meals:

- Can help kickstart and increase the body's own metabolism
- Burn extra calories through thermogenetics
- Aids the body in digestion
- Increases the feeling of fullness before meals
- Adds essential nutrients to the body that, when depleted, can inhibit proper function of the body, including digestion and the body's ability to properly burn calories

Apple cider vinegar is the vinegar-of-choice for weight loss due to its particular makeup. Because this type of vinegar is made up of dozens of nutrients and compounds not found in other types of vinegar, it is thought to have a greater potential for weight loss. Many people swear by the simple extra kick their body received from the apple cider vinegar tonic recipes that follow.

In a nutshell, successful weight loss happens most easily when we eat a well balanced diet consisting of as many whole, natural foods as possible, exercise regularly (even if it is just taking a daily stroll around the neighborhood or working in the flower garden), and seeing if your body reacts by trying an extra boost from apple cider vinegar!

Daily Tonic
Combine 2 teaspoonfuls of apple cider vinegar with 1 teaspoon honey and 1 glass of water. Consume this once a day.

Vinegar Before Meals
To receive the greatest benefit from this, try drinking 10 to 20 minutes before mealtime. Just stir 1 teaspoon apple cider vinegar into 1 cup of water and enjoy!

Vinegar Before Meals Alternative
The addition of honey to this recipe makes it more palatable if the taste of vinegar is too strong. Just combine 1 teaspoon apple cider vinegar with 1 teaspoon honey in a cup of water, and drink 10 to 20 minutes before each mealtime for best results.

A Thank You Note
from Emily!

Thank you, once again, dear reader, for your continued interest in natural healing ways. It has been a pleasure to bring you this book, and all its exciting uses for vinegar.

If you have a natural healing remedy, unique or special cleaning method or fun, old-time recipe that your family has used, would you consider sharing it with other readers just like yourself? If I use it in one of my upcoming books, you will receive a free copy of the book upon printing.

Please fill out the form that follows and mail it back to me. If the form is missing or isn't available, feel free to use a sheet of paper and mail your ideas in to us.

Thank you again, and my warmest wishes for a long, healthy, happy life.

Emily Thacker

Emily, here is one of my favorite uses for vinegar:

_____

_____

_____

Can we use your name and city when crediting this remedy in the book?

❑ Yes, please credit this remedy to:

_____

_____

❑ No, please use my remedy, but do not use my name in the book.

Either way, yes or no, if I use your remedy, I'll send you a free copy of the new edition of home remedies.

Your remedy can be one which uses vinegar, or simply one that you feel others would like to know about.

My favorite chapter in "*Vinegar Prescription*" is:

_____

The most helpful remedy I appreciated in "*Vinegar Prescription*" is:

_____

_____

What I liked best about "*Vinegar Prescription*" is:

_____

_____

Would you be interested in hearing about my new cookbook when it becomes available?

_____

My name and mailing address is:

_____

_____

If you have any comments or experiences to add to the information you've read in this collection, or if you have information for subsequent editions, please address your letters to:

Emily Thacker
PO Box 980
Hartville, OH 44632

Preferred Customer Reorder Form

Order this...	If you want a book on...	Cost...	Number of Copies...
Amish Vinegar Secrets	No one knows natural healing and prevention better than the AMISH! This must-read reveals generations worth of all-natural healing remedies and potent cleaning techniques using everyday household vinegar.	$9.95	
The Vinegar Anniversary Book	Completely updated with the latest research and brand new remedies and uses for apple cider vinegar. Handsome coffee table collector's edition you'll be proud to display.	$9.95	
The Magic of Hydrogen Peroxide	An Ounce of Hydrogen Peroxide is worth a Pound of Cure! Hundreds of health cures, household uses & home remedy uses for hydrogen peroxide contained in this breakthrough volume.	$9.95	
The Magic of Baking Soda	*Plain Old Baking Soda A Drugstore in A Box?* Doctors & researchers have discovered baking soda has amazing healing properties! Over 600 health & Household Hints. *Great Recipes Too!*	$9.95	
Amish Gardening Secrets	You too can learn the special gardening secrets the Amish use to produce huge tomato plants and bountiful harvests. Information packed 800-plus collection for you to tinker with and enjoy.	$9.95	

Any combination of the above $9.95 items qualifies for the following discounts...

	Total NUMBER of $9.95 items	

Order any 2 items for: **$15.95**

Order any 3 items for: **$19.95**

Order any 4 items for: **$24.95**

Order any 5 items for: **$29.95**

Order any 6 items for: **$34.95** and receive 7th item FREE

Any additional items for: **$5 each**

FEATURED SELECTIONS		Total COST of $9.95 items	
The Honey Book	Amazing Honey Remedies to relieve arthritis pain, kill germs, heal infection and much more!	$19.95	
The Cinnamon Book	Research studies have found this amazing spice is loaded with health benefits. Find out how cinnamon can be used in treating common (and not so common) conditions such as diabetes, obesity, arthritis, high cholesterol and a host of other ailments.	$19.95	
Hydrogen Peroxide Formula Guide	FINALLY...No more guesswork! Step-by-step instructions and specific measurements for hundreds of amazing hydrogen peroxide uses. Learn how to use hydrogen peroxide to clean your home, balance pH soil levels, use as a home remedy or beautify your life! It is all here!	$19.95	

Order any 2 or more Featured Selections for only $10 each...

	Postage & Handling	$3.98*
	TOTAL	

90-DAY MONEY-BACK GUARANTEE

***** *Shipping of 10 or more books = $6.96*

Please rush me the items marked above. I understand that I must be completely satisfied or I can return any item within 90 days for a full and prompt refund of my purchase price.

I am enclosing $_____ by: ❑ Check ❑ Money Order (Make checks payable to James Direct Inc)

Charge my credit card Signature _____

Card No. _____ Exp. Date _____

Name _____ Address _____

City _____ State_____ Zip _____

Telephone Number (_____) _____

❑ Yes! I'd like to know about freebies, specials and new products before they are nationally advertised. My email address is: _____

Mail To: **James Direct Inc.** • PO Box 980, Dept. A1434 • Hartville, Ohio 44632
Customer Service (330) 877-0800 • *http://www.jamesdirect.com*

AMISH VINEGAR SECRETS

Learn the Amish way to better health! Studies indicate the Amish have less instances of asthma, cardiovascular disease and some forms of cancer. Learn their secrets to better health using everyday household vinegar to treat common (and not-so-common) illness, prevent sickness before it sets in and have a germ-free household.

THE VINEGAR ANNIVERSARY BOOK

Handsome coffee table edition and brand new information on Mother Nature's Secret Weapon – apple cider vinegar!

THE MAGIC OF HYDROGEN PEROXIDE

Hundreds of health cures & home remedy uses for hydrogen peroxide. You'll be amazed to see how a little hydrogen peroxide mixed with a pinch of this or that from your cupboard can do everything from relieving chronic pain to making age spots go away! Easy household cleaning formulas too!

THE MAGIC OF BAKING SODA

We all know baking soda works like magic around the house. It cleans, deodorizes & works wonders in the kitchen and in the garden. But did you know it's an effective remedy for allergies, bladder infection, heart disorders... *and MORE!*

AMISH GARDENING SECRETS

There's something for everyone in *Amish Gardening Secrets*. This BIG collection contains over 800 gardening hints, suggestions, time savers and tonics that have been passed down over the years in Amish communities and elsewhere.

THE HONEY BOOK

Each page is packed with healing home remedies and ways to use honey to heal wounds, fight tooth decay, treat burns, fight fatigue, restore energy, ease coughs and even make cancer-fighting drugs more effective. Great recipes too!

THE CINNAMON BOOK

Cinnamon is rich in natural healing properties such as being an anti-oxidant, anti-inflammatory, anti-coagulant, anti-microbial, anti-parasitic, anti-tumor – just to name a few! Find out how cinnamon can be used to fight everything from simple cuts and scrapes to chronic health condition, safely and naturally!

HYDROGEN PEROXIDE FORMULA GUIDE

This unique book lists hundreds of home remedy, gardening and cleaning uses for peroxide along with exact measurements and instructions for each use. No mistakes and no guesswork.

* Each Book has its own FREE Bonus!

All these important books carry our NO-RISK GUARANTEE. Enjoy them for three full months. If you are not 100% satisfied simply return the book(s) for a prompt, "no questions asked" refund!

www.ingramcontent.com/pod-product-compliance
Lightning Source LLC
Chambersburg PA
CBHW060907280326
41934CB00007B/1225